STATISTICAL METHODS FOR COST-EFFECTIVENESS RESEARCH: A GUIDE TO CURRENT ISSUES AND FUTURE DEVELOPMENTS

Edited by Andrew H. Briggs

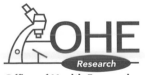

Office of Health Economics

Office of Health Economics
12 Whitehall London SW1A 2DY
www.ohe.org

© November 2003. Office of Health Economics. Price £12.50

ISBN 1 899040 72 2

Office of Health Economics

The Office of Health Economics (OHE) was founded in 1962. Its terms of reference are to:

- commission and undertake research on the economics of health and health care;

- collect and analyse health and health care data from the UK and other countries;

- disseminate the results of this work and stimulate discussion of them and their policy implications.

The OHE is supported by an annual grant from the Association of the British Pharmaceutical Industry and by revenue from sales of its publications, consultancy and commissioned research.

CONTENTS

LIST OF CONTRIBUTORS

Dr Andrew H. Briggs
Health Economics Research Centre, University of Oxford, England

Dr George W. Carides
Merck Research Laboratories, Pennsylvania, USA

Dr John Cook
Merck Research Laboratories, Pennsylvania, USA

Dr Henry Glick
University of Pennsylvania, USA

Professor Daniel F. Heitjan
University of Pennsylvania, and formerly Columbia University, USA

Professor Tony O'Hagan
University of Sheffield, England

Professor Ben Van Hout
University of Utrecht, the Netherlands

Professor Andrew Willan
McMaster University, Canada

Chapter 1
Introduction

ANDREW H. BRIGGS

Health economic evaluation has come of age. There are few industrialised countries that do not now recognise the importance for decision-making of evidence on the cost-effectiveness of interventions. Cost-effectiveness evidence is not a formal regulatory requirement in the licensing of new medications. But it is clear that bodies such as the National Institute for Clinical Excellence (NICE) in the UK, the Canadian Coordinating Office for Health Technology Assessment (CCHOTA) and the Pharmaceutical Benefits Advisory Committee (PBAC) in Australia are part of a general trend towards the direct use of cost-effectiveness information to decide on health care interventions for routine clinical practice.

In the early days, many health economic evaluations proceeded by synthesising the results of published studies available in the literature. But as a consequence of the increased interest in cost-effectiveness evidence, it is now common to find economic variables collected prospectively alongside clinical trials.

The existence of patient-level data on both costs and effects of interventions generated by such studies has naturally led to an increased interest in the use of statistical methods to analyse the data. While many of the issues faced in analysing cost-effectiveness data are similar to those when analysing clinical data, cost-effectiveness analysis generates a number of particular challenges that mean new methods have had to be developed.

Methodological development over the last decade has been rapid, with many alternative techniques having been suggested for economic evaluation, not all of which have stood the test of time. As a result, the recent literature on the topic of statistical methods for cost-effectiveness analysis is something of a minefield, with the state of the art such that what was once considered acceptable in terms of analysis may no longer be considered appropriate. Furthermore, the recent nature of many developments means that not all have yet been captured in popular textbooks in this area.

Chapter 2
Analysing cost-effectiveness trials: net benefits

ANDREW WILLAN

This paper is concerned with some of the statistical approaches that are available for statistical cost-effectiveness analysis when comparing two groups. The model I am going to use is a randomised clinical trial but the approach is pretty much the same for any two groups, whether randomised or not. The aim is to provide a brief overview of the work that has been done in this area for the last five or six years. Much of the technical detail will be omitted but can be found in the literature. Instead the focus will be on the development of, and the intuition behind, the methods.

Consider a clinical trial in which patients are randomised between two therapies: standard (S) and treatment (T). Let e_{ji} and c_{ji} be measures of effectiveness and cost on the ith patient of the jth therapy: $j=S,T$; $i=1,2,...n_j$; and n_j is the respective sample size. The expectation of e_{ji} is denoted by μ_j and the expectation of c_{ji} is denoted by v_j. The variance structure is given by

$$V\begin{pmatrix} e_{ji} \\ c_{ji} \end{pmatrix} = \Sigma_j = \begin{pmatrix} \sigma_j^2 & \rho_j\sigma_j\omega_j \\ \rho_j\sigma_j\omega_j & \omega_j^2 \end{pmatrix}$$

where σ_j^2 is the variance of the effects, ω_j^2 the variance in costs, and ρ_j the correlation coefficient between costs and effects for the jth therapy.

What we are really interested in is estimating the expected increase in effectiveness using treatment rather than standard: $\Delta_e = \mu_T - \mu_S$, and the expected increase in costs using treatment rather than standard: $\Delta_c = v_T - v_S$. We have to make a few assumptions about these estimates.

Our job is to find unbiased estimates for the difference in effect and the difference in costs. We are going to assume when we have these estimates that that they are normally distributed and unbiased, so that the expected values are the true parameters. We are interested in estimating the variances of each difference and the covariance between them. Thus there are five things to estimate. The first two are the difference in effects and the difference in costs. But you also have to take into account the respective variances of the effect and cost differences and the covariance between them. What follows is pretty straight forward if you keep in mind that we are simply trying to estimate these five things.

When we have estimated those five things we can calculate an incremental cost-effectiveness ratio (ICER). This is defined simply as the change in the cost over the change in effect: $ICER = \Delta_c / \Delta_e$. Thus it measures the additional costs of achieving an extra unit of effectiveness by using treatment rather than standard.

You could use a net benefit approach where you take the difference in effects multiplied by what we call the willingness to pay (λ) to convert that into a monetary benefit

$$b(\lambda) = \lambda \cdot \Delta_e / \Delta_c$$

The net benefit is the improvement in health multiplied by what we think that improvement is worth, less the additional cost; so net benefit just measures in dollars the added benefit of using treatment over standard for each patient.

The benefit of this formulation of net benefit (you may have seen some others) is that where you can have more than one measure of effectiveness, you can string them all out with a specific willingness to pay for each particular aspect of effectiveness measured. For example, where there are k different effects measured in a clinical trial, then providing that we can specify k different willingness to pay values for those effects, λ_k, then it is straightforward to generate the net benefit as

$$b(\lambda_1, \lambda_2 \dots, \lambda_k) = \Delta_{e1} \lambda_1 + \Delta_{e2} \lambda_2 + \dots + \Delta_{ek} \lambda_k - \Delta_c$$

You might also want to do a cost-minimisation analysis where you are either assuming that there is no difference in effects, which is not usually a good assumption, or you just do not care about the difference in effects. You would then just be looking at the difference in cost, which is minus net benefit for $\lambda=0$. That is, we consider cost-minimisation analysis as a special case of the net benefit approach.

Consider Figure 2.1, which shows net benefit as a function of the willingness to pay for health gain measured in quality adjusted life years (QALYs), λ. The slope of the line is the difference in effects. Where the line meets the vertical axis is (minus) the difference in costs, and where it crosses the horizontal axis is the ICER (i.e. where net benefit is zero). Thus from this simple plot you can see the net benefit for every value of λ, the ICER, the difference in costs and the difference in effects. Our job is to estimate these things from the data.

Figure 2.1 **Parameters of interest**

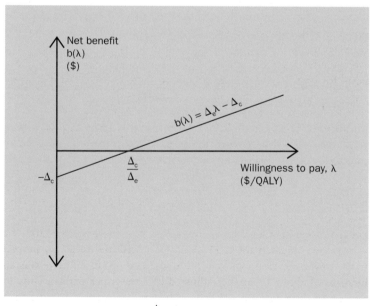

Note that $b(0) = -\Delta_c$ and $b\left(\dfrac{\Delta_c}{\Delta_e}\right) = 0$

Now let us consider an example to illustrate the approach. In a study there are 161 patients who have end stage prostate cancer. They are just being treated palliatively, which for the standard care arm of the trial is prednisone alone and in the treatment arm of the trial is mitoxantrone added to the prednisone. There was no difference in survival between the groups. We went back and obtained the cost data for 114 of the patients in the three larger centres involved in the clinical trial and quality-adjusted the survival using quality of life question C30 from the European Organisation for Research and Treatment of Cancer (EORTC) questionnaire. It was not designed to be used in this way but we wanted to somehow compensate for the fact that there was potentially a large difference in the quality of life between the two study arms.

Within 18 months all 161 patients had died, so there was no censoring of the data. When there is no censoring you can just use sample means and variances to estimate the five parameters required for cost-effectiveness analysis. To estimate the difference in effects between the two arms of the trial you just take the difference in the average effects, because there is no censoring. You can do exactly the same for cost. The variances are obtained from the between-patient sample estimates of variance, which are then divided by the sample size to convert to a variance of a mean. Thus when there is no censoring it is very straightforward to estimate the five parameters; and once you have estimated the five parameters it is very straightforward to estimate cost-effectiveness.

It turns out that the average cost per person in the treatment group was $27,300 compared to $29,000 in the standard group, so there was a saving of about $1,700 (all currency amounts in this chapter are expressed in Canadian dollars). When we quality-adjusted the survival we obtained about 41 quality-adjusted life weeks per person in the treatment group and 28 in the standard group, so there was an increase of about 13 quality-adjusted life weeks per person. Thus in this a case there is a win-win situation: the treatment is better and it costs less. The ICER is -$134 per quality of life week saved.

Figure 2.2 **Problems with ICERS**

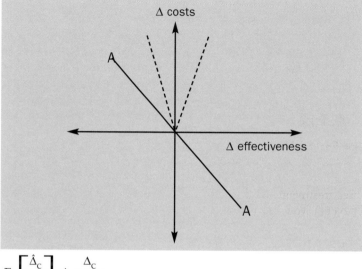

$$E\left[\frac{\hat{\Delta}_c}{\hat{\Delta}_e}\right] \neq \frac{\Delta_c}{\Delta_e}$$

However, there are a lot of problems with using ICERs:

- the first is that you cannot estimate it without bias. This is not a huge problem as the bias rapidly approaches zero as the sample size increases, but nevertheless people sometimes highlight that as a weakness;

- another issue is that the confidence intervals can include an undefined value. Figure 2.2 shows a cost-effectiveness plane. Consider the confidence interval represented by the two broken lines. This interval includes the vertical axis where effect is zero, which gives an undefined value for the ICER;

- furthermore, the upper limit is negative and the lower limit is positive, which, without at least plotting it on the cost-effectiveness plane, is a little hard to explain;

- another problem is that ICERs can have exactly the same value but mean two different things. Consider the (negative) ICER value represented by the line AA on Figure 2.2. Points on this line in the win-win (south-east) quadrant favour the new treatment, while points in the lose-lose (north-west) quadrant favour the existing treatment. But points on this line have exactly the same ICER in both quadrants;

- confidence intervals can be undefined, if your data are too close to the origin so that you really cannot define a confidence interval for ICER.

One final problem with ICERs, which really got me concerned, is that they are not properly ordered outside the trade-off quadrants. Let me illustrate what I mean by that. Consider Figure 2.3, which shows three treatments compared to a standard treatment. With treatment one (T1) you get two extra units of effectiveness relative to the

Figure 2.3 **ICERs are not properly ordered outside trade-off quadrants**

	Effect. (years)	Cost ($1000s)	
T1	5	8	
T2	7	6	
T3	7	8	
S	3	10	ICER
Δ1	2	-2	-1
Δ2	4	-4	1
Δ3	4	-2	-0.5

standard treatment (S) and you save $2,000. With treatment two (T2) you get four extra units of effectiveness and save $4,000. Treatment two is therefore a lot better than treatment one, but the ICER is exactly the same, -1, in each case. Treatment three saves about the same amount of money as treatment one but has twice as much improvement in effectiveness, yet its ICER is actually larger than for treatment one, -0.5>-1. It is therefore meaningless to talk about a confidence interval over a range of values that are not properly ordered: a confidence interval is, strictly speaking, an ordering.

As explained earlier, we can instead conduct our analysis in terms of net benefit. We can do an equivalent analysis either in terms of net monetary benefit (Tambour et al. 1998) or net health benefit (Stinnett and Mullahy 1998). They will both lead to exactly the same results. Essentially what we are looking for is to see if net benefit is positive, which indicates that treatment is cost-effective. My personal preference is to analyse net monetary benefit: it is a linear function of

Figure 2.4 **Net benefit**

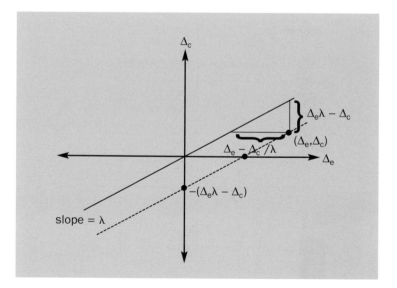

λ (see Figure 2.1); I find it easier to talk about net benefits in terms of dollars; plus it allows for more than one type of measure of effectiveness as described above.

How does net benefit relate to the cost-effectiveness plane? Consider the cost-effectiveness plane shown in Figure 2.4. If you divide the plane by a straight line through the origin with slope equal to λ, all those points above this line have negative net benefit (favouring existing treatment) and all the points below this line have positive net benefit (favouring the new treatment). Consider the point (Δ_e, Δ_c): the vertical distance between that point and the line through the origin with slope λ is the net benefit in monetary terms; the horizontal distance between that point and the same line is the net-benefit in terms of health. If you draw a straight line through the point (Δ_e, Δ_c) parallel to the line through the origin (i.e. also with slope λ) and project it onto the horizontal axis, then this is also equal to the net benefit in terms of effectiveness. Continuing the projection to the vertical axis gives negative net-benefit in monetary terms. So the presentation of results on the cost-effectiveness plane gives a little more information than you might imagine.

Figure 2.5 **Net benefit is properly ordered**

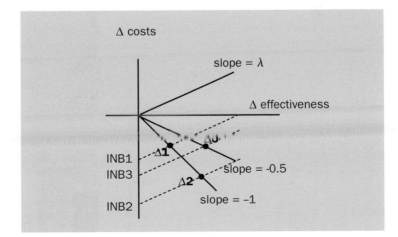

Now consider Figure 2.5, which returns to the example in Figure 2.3 where there was the conflict with respect to the way we thought treatments should be ordered in terms of the ICER. Now let us choose a value for λ and plot a line with this slope that passes through each of the points. If you project these lines back to the vertical axis, you will notice that the incremental net benefit for treatment two (INB2) is the greatest, followed by that of treatment three, and treatment one has the smallest net benefit. Thus, net benefit orders the treatments in the same way we thought they should be ordered in the first place. All we have done is project back to the vertical axis using the slope λ, representing the willingness to pay for effectiveness.

How do we do an analysis with net benefit? We really want to test the hypothesis that net benefit is negative and reject it if we can, in which case we will adopt treatment over standard. We have seen how to estimate net benefit: it is simply λ multiplied by our estimate for the difference in effects, minus the difference in costs

$$\hat{b}(\lambda) = \lambda \cdot \hat{\Delta}_e - \hat{\Delta}_c$$

You can obtain the variance for net benefit as a simple combination of the estimates for the variances and the covariance of the incremental effects and costs

$$\mathrm{var}\big(\hat{b}(\lambda)\big) = \lambda^2 \cdot \mathrm{var}\big(\hat{\Delta}_e\big) + \mathrm{var}\big(\hat{\Delta}_c\big) - 2\lambda \cdot \mathrm{cov}\big(\hat{\Delta}_e, \hat{\Delta}_c\big)$$

Again, you can see that we only have to estimate five parameters: the difference in costs, the difference in effects, the variances in each, plus the covariance between them. Where we have complete data this can be done with introductory level statistics which we are all familiar with. To test the hypothesis that net benefit is negative we can use a z-test: we simply take the estimated net benefit and divide it by the square root of the variance and compare it to the critical value from the normal distribution. More likely, we would want to simply estimate uncertainty by constructing confidence intervals for many different values of λ.

Figure 2.6 shows this analysis for the prostate cancer example I referred to earlier. The middle line is the estimated net benefit as a function of the willingness to pay, λ, for an extra quality-adjusted life week (QALW). The slope of the line is positive because we have observed an increase in effectiveness when switching from standard therapy to the new treatment. Since the net benefit line hits the vertical axis at a positive value we know that new treatment is associated with reduced cost: it hits the vertical axis at $-\Delta_c$, $1,700, so the difference in cost (treatment cost minus standard cost) is $-$1,700. The point at which the net-benefit line hits the horizontal axis gives the ICER, which is negative for this example, -$134. Figure 2.6 also shows confidence intervals around the net benefit for every value of λ. Where these intervals cross the vertical axis gives the confidence interval for the cost difference. Where the net benefit intervals cross the horizontal axis is the confidence interval for the ICER, which is identical to the Fieller theorem solution. If you are really brave and are prepared to say 'I think it's worth paying $1,500 for a quality adjusted life week', we can get an estimate of the net

Figure 2.6 **Net benefit as a function of willingness to pay (λ) – prostate cancer example**

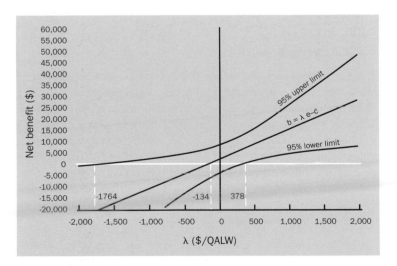

QALW = Quality Adjusted Life Week

benefit and associated confidence interval for that value of λ. So we can do all three analyses on a single graph and all we have had to use is introductory statistics.

This all sounds too good to be true and of course it is, because in almost all cases except for when all the patients die or you follow them for as long as the period of interest, you are going to have censored data. Censored data typically occur because, even if patients are not lost to follow-up, patients randomised in the last few years of the trial will not be followed for the entire duration of interest. For example the period of interest may be five years but you may want to do an analysis two years after the last patient was randomised.

This is where the analysis starts to become unwieldy. George Carides covers a number of procedures for handling censored cost data in Chapter 6, but I will introduce here an example using censored data. Six hundred patients at risk of having a cardiac arrest were randomised between their current medical treatment (amiodarone) and an implanted cardioverter defibrillator (ICD). For the economic analysis, the measure of effectiveness was mean survival, and we restricted our time period to a fixed period after randomisation. This means that we assumed that the survival curves and the rates at which patients accumulate cost after this period are the same in both groups, or at least negligibly different.

If you want to estimate mean survival and you do not have complete follow-up, then you just need the area under the survival curve, which can be estimated simply using the standard Kaplan-Meier estimates. A Kaplan-Meier survival curve is flat and takes a drop every time there is a death; to get the mean survival for each treatment group, you simply have to add up all the rectangles defined at the points that someone dies. Of course, we also need an estimate of the variance for the mean survival in each group and although the formula for the variance is pretty ugly, it is a standard method and can be found in any medical statistics book.

The problem is that if you have cost data and they are censored, you cannot use this standard Kaplan-Meier method directly. That is, you cannot simply use cost to death instead of time to death because you have what we call informative censoring and this leads to positively biased estimates. Instead, you have to use the Lin method (Lin et al. 1997) as discussed by George Carides in Chapter 6. You divide the time from entry into the study into increments (which do not have to be equally spaced) and calculate the mean cost for that interval for patients who were not censored within the interval. Most of the trials I have been involved with have cost histories, so typically we record when the cost is incurred. In order to calculate the mean cost for each treatment group, within each time interval, you just include all the patients that enter the time period and were not censored – they might have died during that time period, but they were not censored during that time period – and calculate their average costs for that interval.

To obtain the overall cost estimate for the patient group, we multiply the mean cost during each interval by the proportion of patients alive at the beginning of the interval and then sum across all intervals. This is our estimate of expected cost. Unfortunately, the variance expression for this estimate of cost is rather messy and the covariance expression is even worse – the expressions themselves can be found in Willan and Lin 2001. The point is that we are trying to estimate the same five things as before: the difference in effects, the difference in costs, the variances of those estimates and their covariance. The expressions are more complex now, but the approach is the same.

Having estimated these five things for the ICD study in the presence of censoring, we can again estimate net benefit and construct a confidence interval, all as a function of willingness to pay for additional years of life, λ. This is presented in Figure 2.7, which is limited to positive values of λ, since negative values do not really make sense. Again the net benefit line has a positive slope, so you know that the new treatment improves effectiveness. The net benefit line hits the cost axis at a negative value (i.e. a negative cost saving), so treatment increases costs, and where it crosses the horizontal axis is the ICER, an estimated $188,500 per life year gained (note, no quality adjustment).

Figure 2.7 **Net benefit as a function of willingness to pay (λ)
– for CIDS example**

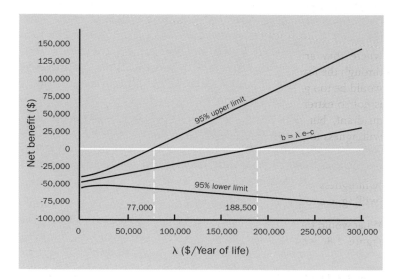

Along the vertical axis we can look at a cost minimisation analysis, not that it would make sense in this case, but you can estimate the difference in cost together with a confidence interval. Where the upper limit of net benefit crosses the horizontal axis we get the lower limit of the ICER, an estimate of $77,000 per life-year gained. The lower limit of net benefit never actually reaches the horizontal axis and that just means that there is no limit to what the extra cost of a life year could be, and this is reflected in a confidence interval for the ICER where the upper limit is inside the lose-lose (north west) quadrant of the cost-effectiveness plane.

Up to now we have been assuming a constant trade off between costs and effects, λ, represented by the straight line on the cost-effectiveness plane. What this means is that if there were a reduction in effectiveness, we would want to be compensated at the same rate as we are willing to pay for health gain in the north-east quadrant. However, it is common for people to say that in order to give up something that you already have you need to be compensated more than you would be willing to pay for it in the first place. Some people even go so far as to suggest that when the line representing this trade-off between costs and effects hits the vertical axis it becomes vertical itself. In other words, there are no circumstances where they are willing to give up effectiveness – this might be through the fear of being sued or because the perceived political costs would be too great or whatever. However, let us assume that the effect is not so extreme, and that there is some trade off in the south-west quadrant, but that it is at a greater level than when considering willingness to pay for increased effectiveness. That is, we would need greater compensation to give up something we already have than we would be willing to pay for it in the first place. In other words, the 'willingness to accept (WTA)' has a greater magnitude than the 'willingness to pay (WTP)'.

What would this mean for our analysis of cost-effectiveness? Consider Figure 2.8, which shows ellipses representing the joint density of

Figure 2.8 **Net benefit when WTA > WTP (WTA = γWTP; γ>1)**

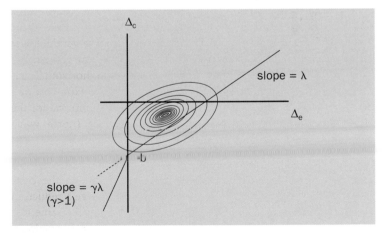

$$\int\limits_{-\infty}^{0}\int\limits_{\lambda\gamma e\text{-}b}^{\infty}f(e,c)dcde +\int\limits_{0}^{\infty}\int\limits_{\lambda e\text{-}b}^{\infty}f(e,c)dcde$$

Figure 2.9 **Acceptability curve when WTA > WTP**
(WTA = γWTP; γ>1)

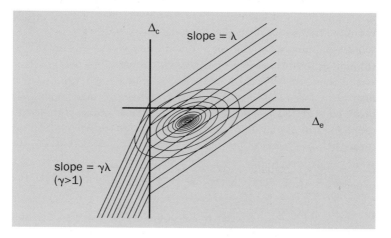

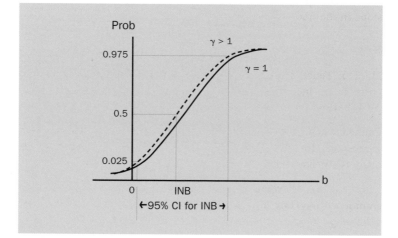

$$\int\limits_{-\infty}^{0}\int\limits_{\lambda\gamma e-b}^{\infty}f(e,c)dcde + \int\limits_{0}^{\infty}\int\limits_{\lambda e-b}^{\infty}f(e,c)dcde$$

costs and effects on the cost-effectiveness plane. If the willingness to accept is γ times greater than the willingness to pay, then the line representing our decision rule will have a kink at the origin, since the slope will be different in the two trade-off quadrants. The slope will be λ in the north-east and south-east quadrants and $\gamma\lambda$ in the south-west quadrant. When we look at the area above this kinked line (indicating treatment is not cost-effective), it has to include a greater area than if we had simply projected a straight line with slope λ through both quadrants. Therefore, my estimate of incremental net benefit will decrease and the confidence interval limits will actually move towards the origin, all because we are including more area, more probability, above the line.

In terms of acceptability curves, which show the probability that net benefits are positive as a function of λ, the effect of introducing a kink at the origin can be seen in Figure 2.9. The acceptability curve for $\gamma > 1$ (i.e. when willingness to accept, WTA, is greater than willingness to pay, WTP) lies above that for the case where $\gamma = 1$, which corresponds to the standard approach of assuming the same slope in the trade-off quadrants.

REFERENCES

Lin, D.Y., Feuer, E.J., Etzioni, R. and Wax, Y. 1997, 'Estimating medical costs from incomplete follow-up data', Biometrics, vol.53, no.2, pp.419-434.

Stinnett, A. A. and Mullahy, J. 1998, 'Net health benefits: a new framework for the analysis of uncertainty in cost-effectiveness analysis', Medical Decision Making, vol.18, no.2, Suppl, pp.S68-S80.

Tambour, M., Zethraeus, N. and Johannesson, M. 1998, 'A note on confidence intervals in cost-effectiveness analysis', International Journal of Technology Assessment in Health Care, vol.14, no.3, pp.467-471.

Willan, A. R. and Lin, D. Y. 2001, 'Incremental net benefit in randomized clinical trials', Statistics in Medicine, vol.20, no.11, pp.1563-1574.

Chapter 3
Sample size calculations for cost-effectiveness studies

BEN VAN HOUT

This paper concerns power calculations, and will include first the simple theory of power calculations for effectiveness only (i.e. just one dimension). I will then move on to consider two dimensions: both costs and effects. Finally, I consider practical applications of the methods.

I start with the familiar cost-effectiveness plane. The difference in effectiveness is on the horizontal axis and the difference of cost is on the vertical axis. In an evaluation of a new treatment, if we end up in the south-east quadrant where treatment dominates, then we are very happy since we have more effectiveness at less cost. If we end up in the north-west quadrant it is very sad since the new treatment is clearly no good. If we end up in the southwest or northeast quadrants then there is a trade-off to be made and this is where the health economist makes a living.

In terms of power, when we are planning a trial we are concerned about how many patients we need to include in it to be able to detect a reasonable treatment effect. We have a type one error α, the chance of falsely rejecting the null hypothesis of no difference between the treatments, and a type two error β, the chance that we fail to reject the null hypothesis when a treatment effect exists. The power is defined as $1-\beta$, the chance that we correctly reject the null hypothesis.

What we need are expectations about the average effectiveness and the variance of the average effectiveness. We must first specify our null hypothesis, and we may indeed have a number of null hypotheses we wish to consider:

- a two-sided hypothesis that treatments are equally effective, such that evidence of a treatment effect in either direction leads us to reject the null;

- a one-sided hypothesis that the new treatment is no better than the existing treatment;

- or an equivalence design where the null hypothesis is that the treatments differ in effectiveness and the aim of the study is to show that this is not the case (within some range of equivalence).

The standard textbook result for the sample size calculation, based on a null hypothesis of equal treatment effects and assuming the same number of patients is to be recruited to each arm of the clinical trial is given by

$$n = \frac{(z_\alpha + z_{2\beta})^2 (\sigma_1^2 + \sigma_2^2)}{(\mu_1 - \mu_2)^2} + \left\{ \frac{1}{|\mu_1 - \mu_2|} \right\}$$

where z is the critical value from the normal distribution to give the appropriate type I and type II error rates, μ_t is the expected effectiveness and σ_t^2 the variance for the treatment groups $t = 1, 2$.

For example, assume a 20% event rate when there is no treatment, i.e. we expect that patients would come back about 20% of the time, and that the event rate would decrease to 10% with treatment, i.e. a 50% reduction in the event rate. We want to reject a null hypothesis if α is smaller than 0.05, and we want the power to be at least 0.8. Then the sample size needs to be at least 290 in each arm of the trial.

Using this formula and the assumption of asymptotic normality is just one way to find a solution to the sample size problem. An alternative approach would be to use simulation in order to examine the power of any particular sample size. This is particularly useful when preparing for a randomised clinical trial. The approach is to simulate a trial with, for example, 1,000 patients. Given the expected event rates as before – 90% of patients event-free with treatment and 80% event-free without – you run the simulation 10,000 times, say, and you check for each sample size whether the null hypothesis is rejected in each trial and record the result. The proportion of the 10,000 trials in which the null hypothesis is not rejected then gives the power for the given sample size. Now it is a simple case of plotting the power as a function of the sample size, which leads you to the numbers of patients required. So it is not necessary to use a formula and parametric assumptions given the power of desktop computers to undertake very large numbers of simulations in a short time.

Figure 3.1 shows the results of just such a simulation presenting power as a function of the number of subjects. From the figure we see that if we want a power of about 90% then we need about 290 patients. If we were to use the standard mathematical formula then the curve generated falls right on top of the curve estimated through the simulation experiment in Figure 3.1.

So far I have presented the one-dimensional case of an effectiveness evaluation only, to show how the standard approach works. I now extend the problem to the two-dimensional case of cost-effectiveness evaluation. Typically now we are considering cost-effectiveness analyses of drugs alongside clinical trials, and due to the vested interests of the pharmaceutical industry there is much regulation concerning the design and analysis of such trials. In particular, there will be very well defined protocols and analysis plans. Definitions of

Figure 3.1 **Power as a function of the number of subjects, for effectiveness only**

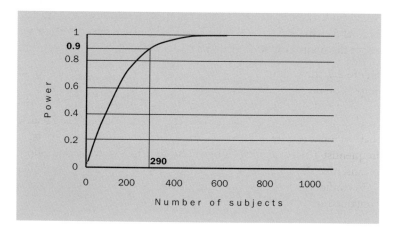

26

cost, of effect and of cost-effectiveness will already be in the trial protocol. We have a say in how we are going to collect the data, what statistical methods will be used, and how the results will be presented.

One point I would like to stress here is that we act as if we know the unit costs. Unit costs used to value the resource use observed in clinical trials tend to be treated as if they are fixed and known. We typically act as if there is no uncertainty surrounding cost calculations, whereas in my view there is considerable uncertainty.

With this point in mind, I turn to the problem of representing uncertainty in the two-dimensional case where we are looking at both costs and effects. We know, from the central limit theorem, that we can assume that average costs and effects are normally distributed. However, we also know that the cost-effectiveness ratio itself may not have a finite expectation or a finite variance since we know that the ratio of two standard normal distributions (the Cauchy distribution) does not have a finite expectation or a finite variance. We also know that 95% confidence limits for the cost-effectiveness ratio will probably not be symmetrically distributed, so for an estimated cost-effectiveness ratio of $20,000, the confidence limits may turn out to be $10,000 to $50,000.

There are two real solutions to the problem of estimating confidence limits for cost-effectiveness ratios. Either we can assume a bivariate normal distribution (which is essentially the Fieller approach); or we adopt the bootstrapping approach.

Figure 3.2 shows how I prefer to present cost-effectiveness results: as ellipses on the cost-effectiveness plane. The outer ellipse contains 95% of the probability distribution, and this is the smallest area on the plane that contains with 95% probability both cost and effect. I realise that saying these words makes me a Bayesian. If I want to be a frequentist I need a much longer sentence to say what the ellipse means. Also shown in Figure 3.2 are the rays representing the Fieller 95% confidence limits: 95% of the joint density of costs and effects is contained between the rays.

Figure 3.2 **Confidence ellipses and Fieller limits on the cost-effectivenes plane**

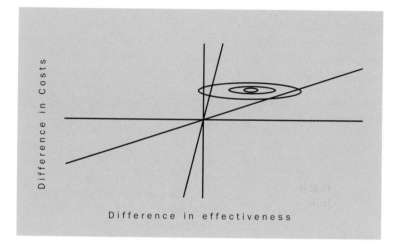

Figure 3.3 **Cost-effectiveness acceptability curve showing the probability that the intervention is cost-effective as a function of the upper limit of acceptability on cost-effectiveness**

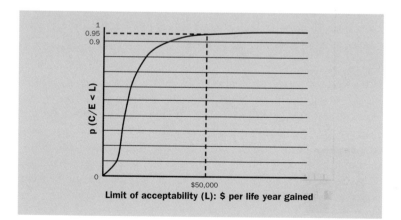

To provide a one-dimensional summary of the cost-effectiveness results we can use an acceptability curve as presented in Figure 3.3. This curve shows for different limits of acceptability – i.e. the highest acceptable cost-effectiveness ratio for decision-makers – how probable it is that the intervention under evaluation is cost-effective. In this illustrative example, if $50,000 per life year gained were judged to be an acceptable limit for decision-making, we have a probability of 0.95 that the intervention lies below this value.

The alternative way to estimate cost-effectiveness confidence limits, bootstrapping, is a non-parametric approach that relies on computing

Figure 3.4 **Distribution of the cost-effectiveness ratio estimated non-parametrically via the boostrap method versus that derived analytically through the assumption of joint normally distibuted costs and effects**

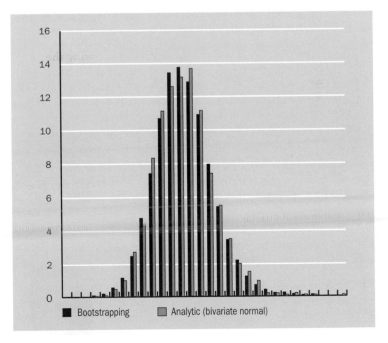

power rather than parametric assumptions. Bootstrap re-samples of the original samples are drawn from the trial data (with replacement) and the original cost-effectiveness calculation is undertaken for this re-sample. The process is then repeated many (say 10,000) times. The frequency distribution of the bootstrapped cost-effectiveness ratios is then calculated and a bootstrap estimate of the acceptability curve can be produced. Figure 3.4 shows a frequency distribution based on bootstrapping compared to an analytic solution from an analysis of a real life trial in the Netherlands. My colleagues and I have now analysed some 11 or 12 trials using bootstrapping methods, but bootstrapping has never given a different result from that which we would have generated using the bivariate normal assumption.

Now that we have considered how cost-effectiveness results from clinical trials are analysed, we can return to the issue of power and sample size in cost-effectiveness studies. Again, we need a null hypothesis (to be rejected); we need a test statistic (as introduced); and we need expectations about the average costs and effects with and without treatment; the variances of costs and effects with and without treatment; and an estimate of the covariance between costs and effects.

There may be several different null hypotheses that could be formulated. One might be that you are interested in both effectiveness and cost-effectiveness. In other words, the null hypothesis would be that the intervention is neither effective nor cost-effective. Alternatively, the null hypothesis might be that the intervention is not cost-effective relative to a particular value of the acceptable limit on cost-effectiveness (e.g. $50,000 per life year gained). Or it might be the case that you would want to use different cost-effectiveness criteria in the north-east and south-west quadrants reflecting the fact that while it may be acceptable to implement a new treatment at $50,000 per life year gained it may only be acceptable to deny a currently provided treatment at $100,000 per life year foregone.

The use of a constant acceptable limit across the quadrants in the cost-effectiveness plane corresponds to the net benefit approach. This is probably the more appropriate formulation, as others have argued. While we do have difficulties with changing from an existing treatment when the replacement is less effective than the existing treatment, albeit less costly, it may be appropriate to consider this issue. However, to date it is not clear that we know the relative trade-offs in the different quadrants, and purely in terms of economic efficiency, the values should really be the same in the north-east as in the south-west quadrant. Until future work clarifies this issue, I will stick with equal acceptable limits in the two quadrants, corresponding to net-benefits.

So to approach the sample size problem in cost-effectiveness we can either look for an appropriate formula in the literature or we can base our calculations on a simulation experiment. For example, Briggs and Gray (1998) present a conservative formula assuming perfect negative covariance between costs and effects. Briggs & Tambour (1998) and Laska et al. (1999), use net benefits to adjust for covariance in their formulae. Alternatively Al et al. (1998) use a simulation approach. It is important to beware of the formulation of the null hypothesis. Some commentators have employed what appear to me to be very strange null hypotheses to generate a sample size formula (e.g. Gardiner et al. 2000).

The simulation approach outlined by Al and colleagues (1998) is essentially the same as that outlined for the one-dimensional case above. You simulate a trial with, say, 1,000 patients, given the expectations of effectiveness with and without treatment (90% and 80% patients being event free respectively). Of course, for the cost-effectiveness problem we also need expectations about costs with and without treatment, and we need expectations about the variance and covariance in the costs and effects. These do not come out of a big hat, so you need either existing information from a pilot study or something else. Simulation may provide the answer.

For example, when we are undertaking trials for cost-effectiveness for cardiovascular disease and interventional cardiology, there are only a few possible events: people have a percutaneous transluminal coronary angioplasty (PTCA) and they might come back for a re-PTCA, they might have bypass surgery, they might have a myocardial infarction, and they might die. These are the only things that can happen to these patients within a time span of two to three years. So, as an example, we can take the cost of an event, modelled say as a log normal distribution with mean 5.9 and standard deviation 1, and apply this to the event rate and add in the cost of treatment for those patients in the treatment arm plus a background cost (say the same lognormal distribution). Overall this generates an expected cost per event avoided of $2,000. By simulating this process we can also generate an estimate of the covariance between costs and effects, and we get more pronounced estimates of the variance of costs and effects.

Applying the simulation method to the estimated costs, effects, variance and covariance allows you to generate a power graph. Figure 3.5 presents the power as a function of the number of subjects for both the cost-effectiveness and the effectiveness only studies. It is clear that to reach the same power in a cost-effectiveness study needs more patients than when studying effectiveness alone. In this illustrative example, for 90% power we would probably need something like 700 or 800 patients for the cost-effectiveness study, compared with just 290 patients to study effectiveness alone.

Figure 3.5 **Power as a function of sample size for a study of effectiveness only and for a study of cost-effectiveness**

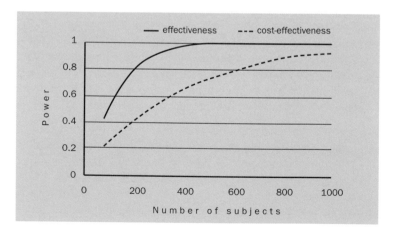

The number of patients needed in a trial for the cost-effectiveness study is a function of a number of different factors. The numbers required in the study increase the lower is the acceptable cost-effectiveness ratio used for decision-making, since then the smaller you want your ellipse to be and so the more observations you need. The numbers also increase the smaller the (positive) difference in effects, the higher the (negative) difference in costs, the higher the variances, and the more negative the correlation between costs and effects.

It is rare for health economists to be asked to contribute to the power calculations of the studies they become involved with and I suspect that at the time of writing I am one of the few people to have done a real-life power calculation that actually informed the design of a cost-effectiveness analysis alongside a clinical trial. The ARTS trial was undertaken to compare bypass surgery with stenting. We supposed in advance that bypass was going to be better than stenting, however, we also knew that stenting was going to be less expensive. We came to the conclusion that cost-effectiveness analysis might be the most appropriate way of trying to express this. With the assumptions about the price of stenting and the price of bypass surgery, we powered that trial in such a way that we needed fewer observations maybe, than if we had just done an effectiveness trial.

Another thing we realised is that the variance between costs is always rather high, and that might mean that there may be valuable information from earlier trials that we were ignoring. For example, if we do a trial comparing stenting with PTCA, and we know a lot more about PTCA because we have all those observations from the past, to do a trial which ignores that previous knowledge seems rather foolish.

When there is existing information which you want to incorporate, then Bayesian methods seem the natural way to go. My understanding is that there is a natural correspondence between the frequentist approach and Bayesian methods using uninformative priors. But we wanted to know what would happen if we tried to use informative prior information. We tried specifying our prior beliefs and using these in the power calculation, but we got into a lot of difficulties. It turned out that the analysis was very sensitive to the choice of prior and this made us very uncomfortable, since it gave the impression that by simply changing our priors slightly we could tailor the result to whatever we wanted. The way I think we should go with the Bayesian approach is to model the whole process using the sorts of decision analytic models we have been using for the last 20 years, but putting in a probabilistic component to the input parameters. The outputs of these models look very much like the elliptical joint distributions we expect from clinical trials.

Turning now from theory to practical application of sample size calculations, my experience has been that sample size calculations often proceed along the following lines. Start by assuming an event rate of 10% and a 10% relative decrease in event rate (i.e. from 10% to 9%). We want to reject the null hypothesis if α is less than 0.05 and we want power of at least 80% to test the difference. This generates a sample size of 14,784. That is a lot of patients and would make the trial too expensive. Let us now assume that we are looking for a 20% decrease in event rate (from 10% to 8%); now the sample size required is about 3,800. This is affordable, but does not give us the status of a really large trial, so we need something a little bigger. Let us therefore assume a 15% decrease in event rate (from 10% to 8.5%) and make the power 90%; now the sample size required is 8,956. That looks like a nice size of trial, so let us stick with that. In other words, all too often the sample size calculation is undertaken backwards: first estimating what sort of sample size is reasonable and then back-solving for the other design parameters.

This illustration was only assuming a one-dimensional effectiveness study. As soon as we include costs, the variance of costs, and the covariance of costs and effects, we open the door to even more potential manipulation. Now when we ask the question of how many subjects are needed for the study, the mathematician will probably say 'hmm', the statistician will give you a nice answer 'maybe between 50 and 600', and the health economist is probably going to say 'how many do you want it to be?'

There are still some problems. I have been involved with the CAPRIE study, which provides an interesting example. This is a large study with over 18,000 patients, to assess the effect of Clopidogrel versus aspirin, and overall it shows a decrease in event rate from 90.22% percent to 89.35%. Clopidogrel costs about $1 and aspirin about 5 cents. In the stroke group we have event rates of 86.61% versus 85.58%, only a slight difference. In the MI group we have event rates of 90.74% versus 91.04%, and in the peripheral artery disease (PAD) group we have 93.33% versus 91.00%. In other words across three events we have one difference that is positive and significant, one that is positive and not statistically significant and one that is negative and not statistically significant. This raises the question of what we should assume about the effect of treatment on event rates: are we to assume a 0.87% reduction in event rate in the whole trial, or should we assume only an effect on the PAD group? I can assure you that clinicians in the Netherlands are not treating the MI patients. Some people are treating PAD cases, and in the stroke patients they do have just a little bit more alternative than just aspirin, so they are not treating them here either. So everybody is looking at the effectiveness and cost-effectiveness of these sub-groups but we still really do not know what the best methodology is for estimating the effectiveness and cost-effectiveness of treatment on these groups. If you want to study sub-groups you have to ensure that the power of each part of the overall study is sufficient, that patient numbers in the sub-groups are high enough.

Overall, I believe that power is a very important concept and one that should be given much more consideration.

My final comment is to make an observation on the debate about whether net benefits are superior to cost-effectiveness ratios. I consider it rather premature to be abandoning cost-effectiveness ratios in favour of net benefits and I will try to explain why. In the Netherlands we have accepted cervical cancer screening which costs about 7,000 per life year gained. We have accepted breast cancer screening which is about 10,000 per life year gained. We have not accepted schemes that are much more intensive with much higher cost-effectiveness ratios, so let us presume that our acceptance limit in the Netherlands is under 20,000 per life year gained. This sort of figure can be gleaned from written reports in the Netherlands. Yet, we have accepted lung transplantation as an appropriate treatment in the Netherlands, which has an estimated cost of about 80,000 per life year gained. We also treat patients with factor 8 and these patients will cost us about 100,000 per year. This is not per life year gained; just to treat them and to make them a little better, costs us 100,000 per year. So in reality we do not have a clue what the maximum acceptance limit is. Therefore, basing an analysis on a statistic that assumes we know what that maximum limit is, seems to me a little strange.

How do I communicate such a statistic to clinicians? If I go to a clinician after he has just been reading that a treatment is associated a 10% decrease in the event rate, and I say that the treatment has negative net-benefits, he is not going to understand. Within many discussions, simply saying that the additional cost per additional event-free survivor is about 10,000 is a lot more useful. Please do not throw away cost-effectiveness ratios just yet!

REFERENCES

Al M.J., Van Hout B.A., Michel B.C. and Rutten F.F. 1998, 'Sample size calculation in economic evaluations', Health Economics, 7(4), pp.327-335.

Briggs A.H. and Gray A.M. 1998, 'Sample size and power calculations for stochastic cost-effectiveness analysis', Medical Decision Making, 18(Suppl.), pp.S81-S92.

Briggs A. and Tambour M. 1998, 'The design and analysis of stochastic cost-effectiveness studies for the evaluation of health care interventions', Swedish Working Papers in Economics, No. 234. [Now published in: Drug Information Journal 2001, 35(4)]

Gardiner J.C., Huebner M., Jetton J. and Bradley C.J. 2000, 'Power and sample assessments for tests of hypotheses on cost-effectiveness ratios', Health Economics, 9(3), pp.227-234.

Laska E.M., Meisner M. and Siegel C. 1999, 'Power and sample size in cost-effectiveness analysis', Medical Decision Making, 19(3), pp.339-343.

Chapter 4
Bayesian methods for analysing cost-effectiveness

DANIEL F. HEITJAN

The essence of cost-effectiveness analysis is that we want somehow to combine cost and effectiveness data together into a rational scheme for allocating resources. In the US the setting is rather different from countries that have national health care systems. Most working people have insurance through their employers, who purchase plans from private insurers, and some individuals purchase health insurance directly from insurance companies. There are insurance systems that are operated or funded by local, state and federal governments, but these are mainly for the poor and elderly. Hence, the consumers of cost-effectiveness analysis in the US are insurance companies, operating in a competitive environment, who are trying to decide what to cover in their health insurance plans. Presumably, the drug and device manufacturers are also keenly interested in what comes out in these analyses because they are selling their products to the insurance companies. The government has a role in this, of course, but probably not as big a role as in Western European countries.

There are two questions of interest here. First, when we are doing cost-effectiveness analysis, what is it that we should be estimating? In statistical terms, what is the estimand? The second question is how to summarise the uncertainty about it. This paper addresses both of these questions.

To fix notation, Figure 4.1 presents the cost-effectiveness plane. On the horizontal axis is the incremental effectiveness, plotting the difference between the effectiveness of treatment one and treatment zero, and on the vertical axis is the difference between the average costs of treatment one and treatment zero.

Considering the question of what to estimate, the concept traditionally used is the incremental cost effectiveness ratio (ICER), defined as the cost difference divided by the effectiveness difference. The context here is clinical trials, which are assumed to give unbiased

Figure 4.1 **The cost-effectiveness plane**

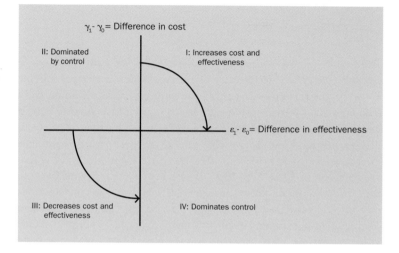

estimates of both the numerator and the denominator of the ICER. Plotting the cost and effectiveness difference pair in the appropriate quadrant of the cost-effectiveness plane, and drawing the ray through that point from the origin, gives the ICER as the slope of that ray. If the new treatment is both more effective and expensive, it lies in the north-east quadrant, and the ICER refers to the cost per additional unit of health that you are purchasing by adopting the new treatment. In the south-west quadrant the ICER represents the savings per unit of health foregone, if the new treatment is used rather than the old one. So in the north-east quadrant you are buying additional units of healthcare at additional cost and in the south-west quadrant you are in a sense selling health, considering adoption of a treatment that is a little less effective but will save a lot of money.

Remember that we are taking the point of view of an insurer operating in a competitive environment, as distinct from that of a patient or a doctor. A key paper here is Karlsson and Johanneson (1996) in which the authors discussed the use of the ICER in a resource allocation mode. Their idealisation of the insurer's problem is that the insurer has a fixed amount of money and has several different populations of policy holders, for instance diabetics, people with heart failure, people with cancer, people with various other combinations of diseases, kids who are healthy, all different kinds of people. For each of the distinct populations there is an array of mutually exclusive treatments available.

The problem for the insurance company is how to allocate its fixed resources among the different diseases so as to provide the optimal amount of benefit for the fixed amount of money that is available. This optimal strategy takes the following steps:

- rank the treatments from least to most effective within each disease category;

- calculate the ICER of each treatment with respect to the next less effective treatment;

- eliminate all the dominated treatments (a treatment is dominated if a combination of the two adjacent treatments is more effective than it is by itself);

- rank the treatments by ICER from lowest to highest.

Using this ranking the insurer will now purchase treatments, starting with those with the lowest ICER, working up the ranking until the budget is exhausted. A lot will depend on how many patients there are requiring each treatment, so in practice there will be a lot of prediction and statistical analysis involved at this stage, but in principle this is how the strategy works. The highest ICER that can be afforded with the fixed budget is what Karlsson and Johanneson call the 'shadow price'. This concept matches up with 'willingness to pay', or λ as it is often known. Even in the US there is plenty of government regulation of health insurance. So there may be States where particular treatments have to be covered, whether the ICER is high or low, in which case such legal and political pressures will distort how this process is going to work. Fundamentally however those are the principles for constructing a rational resource allocation scheme.

So now that we have established what the ICER is and how we would use it if we knew it, we can turn to some very serious issues that arise in estimating the ICER.

The standard approach in the literature, at least implicitly, is to do a clinical trial, estimate the ICER, calculate a confidence interval, and then make the resource allocation decision. Unfortunately, using ICERs in this way leads to a problem of interpretation because so far we have assumed implicitly that the new treatment is always more effective and more costly than the standard, which in reality may not be the case. Specifically, the ICER groups together cost and effectiveness pairs that have totally different meanings, and there is not a single, unambiguous way to rank ICERs.

The point can be illustrated from Figure 4.1. In the north-east quadrant, the more favourable ICERs are those that are closer to the horizontal axis, where the price for purchasing health care is low. In the south-west quadrant, the higher ICERs are more favourable because here you are selling health care rather than buying it, so you want to get the best possible price. So points in the north-east quadrant can be thought of as 'apples' and points in the south-west quadrant as 'oranges'. Any interval for the ICER that fails to distinguish the quadrants is mixing together apples and oranges. It cannot be interpreted.

In the north-east quadrant of Figure 4.1, an arrow going clockwise, towards lower ratios of cost to effect, traces out an arc of improving ICERs. In the south-west quadrant, the arc of better ICERs goes counter-clockwise, toward higher ratios of savings to effect. However, a straight line through the origin shows a value of ICER that is the same (the gradient of the line is the same) in both the north-east and the south-west quadrants. If we rotate this line a little bit clockwise, in the north-east quadrant, that is good, it is a positive move. But that is a negative move in the south-west quadrant, because it moves toward a lower value of return for health foregone. So if all you are given is an interval of ICER values, without knowing which quadrants they are in, then you may be identifying (i.e. grouping together) sets of points in different quadrants that have totally different interpretations.

This is not just an academic point. It is not at all unusual to find in a clinical trial that a new treatment is not significantly more effective, or possibly is even significantly less effective, than the standard treatment. If there is any chance of a negative effect, the ICER and its interval are fundamentally uninterpretable.

In other chapters of this book, Ben Van Hout and Henry Glick both suggest using ellipses and intervals when presenting ICERs. That is fine, because it presents information to enable the ICER to be interpreted. But what has been happening in the literature, at least for some time, is that people present intervals for the ICER as if they were the complete answer. My contention is that such intervals are not meaningful. It is not enough just to show the ICER; you have to say something about which quadrant of the cost-effectiveness plane it is in. Furthermore, as Andy Willan points out in his chapter, for points in the north-west and south-east quadrants we cannot even rank by ICER. At least in the north-east and south-west quadrants we can rank ICERs, but in the other quadrants even points on the same line may not have the same meaning at all.

These are daunting problems. Nevertheless you may decide you still want to estimate ICER, in which case you will encounter some vexing problems of statistical inference. These arise in trying to estimate a ratio parameter. The big issue here is that along the vertical axis of the cost-effectiveness plane (where the effectiveness difference between treatments is zero) the ICER is a discontinuous function of the effectiveness difference. When the effectiveness difference is zero (i.e. the typical null hypothesis in clinical trials) the ICER is infinite. Even worse, as you approach the y-axis from the north-east quadrant the ICER goes off to positive infinity, whereas if you approach from the north-west quadrant the ICER goes off to negative infinity. Moreover, if you have two points that are just on opposite sides of the axis from each other, you would expect them to be similar. But in fact their ICER values are as different as they can be, making it impossible to construct confidence intervals for the ICER. So if you are trying to estimate the ICER and it happens that either the true value or the estimated value of the difference in effectiveness is near zero, you are in this territory and you have problems.

Consider some of the interval estimation methods that people have proposed recently. Over the last few years, health economists have taken a serious interest in summarising uncertainty about ICER. They started by looking at the delta method (Taylor series), the formula used for standard errors in asymptotic statistics. Unfortunately, that formula can fail unless the sample size is very large – much larger than we usually have in clinical trials. The required sample size is larger the closer one gets to the vertical axis, i.e. the smaller the difference in effectiveness. So that method will not work.

The next method considered was Fieller's method, which has advantages and disadvantages. As a confidence set, it works fine no matter where you are in the parameter space, but if the effectiveness difference is not significant, rather than giving you an interval it gives you the outside of an interval, and it can do other pathological things too. So Fieller's method has an undeniable appeal in that it gives you a confidence set that has the correct coverage probability. But it has a strange property in that it produces bizarre confidence sets, which may mean that it should not be used. The problem arises whenever the ICER denominator –the effectiveness difference – is not statistically significant. Because many trials do not give significant results, this behaviour can be a real issue.

Could bootstrapping (i.e. re-sampling from the data) solve this problem? Unfortunately, the problem defeats the bootstrap. It can actually turn it into your enemy. This is not to say that the bootstrap is no good; you still might want to adopt a bootstrap approach as an approximation to something else, or as a way to give robustness to a normality assumption that may be questionable. (The issues that George Carides covers in his chapter are different.) For this ratio estimation problem the bootstrap also suffers from the problem of discontinuity in the ICER estimate.

Table 4.1 is from Heitjan et al. (1999a) showing coverage probabilities – i.e. the performance of a confidence interval in repeated samples – for several methods over a range of true values of the ICER. The rows refer to different combinations of cost and effectiveness differences, and as we move down the table the values

Table 4.1 **Estimated coverage probabilities for various confidence interval methods (%)**

Cases (combinations of cost and effectivenes differences)	Taylor series	Fieller's method	Bootstrap normal	Bootstrap percentile	Bootstrap bias-corrected
'1'	95	94	95	92	90
'2'	92	96	95	97	95
'4'	86	96	94	96	76
'8'	74	96	94	96	64
'16'	56	96	91	86	52

Note: From 400 simulations, $n=50$ per trial arm. The Monte Carlo standard error is no larger than 2.5%.

Source: Heitjan et al. 1999a

get closer to the vertical axis. So as we move from top to bottom in the table, we move towards the troublesome area. The coverage probabilities of the methods refer to the proportion of times, in a hypothetical series of repeated studies, that the interval covers the true value. We want this number to be around 95%.

From the first column, you see that the Taylor series (delta method) interval starts out doing very well when you are far from the vertical axis, but then it falls apart very rapidly as you move toward the vertical axis. Fieller's method works beautifully, in the sense that its coverage probability is right around 95% no matter what the ICER is. The remaining columns are some different versions of the bootstrap approach. Bootstrap normal works pretty well but it starts to deteriorate as you move toward the vertical axis and the same thing happens with the Bootstrap percentile interval. The so-called bias-corrected bootstrap is totally defeated; it is totally fooled by the discontinuity and deteriorates very rapidly. So if you really want to estimate a confidence interval for ICER, there are real problems.

The response has been to accept that if the denominator is near zero then there clearly is a problem, but it is easy to recognise, in which case one would not compute the confidence interval for the ICER. In practice this is a rational approach. The problem, however, is that if you are going to devise a method for constructing an interval, and publish it, then you are under an obligation to describe the method in detail and to ensure that it really is a confidence interval.

In the statistics texts a confidence interval is a *method* for constructing intervals that has the property that the coverage probability is at least some pre-specified value (usually 95%) whatever the value of the underlying parameter. That is, whatever the value of the parameter, the interval will cover it in 95% of hypothetical replications. So if you do not always get an interval, as in the Fieller method, then it is not strictly a confidence interval. Or if the coverage probability is not at least 95%, as with the other methods, then it also is not a confidence interval, and it would be false to say that it was. Now if you acknowledge that there are problems in certain areas, and you provide a method for patching the method up so that the problems do not harm the coverage probability, and you can prove this, then it is acceptable to say you have a confidence interval. But just to leave things up to the judgement of the potential users of the method is in my opinion asking for trouble.

This leads us to the net health benefit approach, which Stinnett and Mullahy (1998) proposed as a way of looking at cost-effectiveness analysis. This is discussed in other chapters, so I merely wish to add a couple of points. First, they proposed the net health benefit as opposed to the net monetary benefit, so they have their number λ in the denominator. Second, the important thing about net benefit is that it is really a utility measurement. Take again the point of view of an insurer. He is trying to maximise the utility that he is offering to his covered population because that is going to give him an edge over his competitors. Because he is trying to maximise the benefit that people are going to get, then the net health benefit is exactly what he wants to look at.

A strategy for selecting treatments would be just to calculate the net health benefit and buy as much as possible of the treatments that offer the greatest net health benefit. A new therapy is adopted if its incremental net health benefit (INHB), compared to the current standard, is positive. The insurer does this for each disease covered. Andy Willan shows us equal-value curves, or isoquants, of INHB: they are simply parallel lines with slope λ in the cost-effectiveness plane. That is, all the points on a line have an INHB of 1, 2, 3, etc. Hence, ICERs in the north-east quadrant do make some sense because they can be ranked unambiguously in that quadrant. Considering Figure 4.1, if the left half of the cost-effectiveness plan is excluded, cost and effectiveness combinations can be ranked by ICER and the result is the same as ranking them by INHB. So if you know which quadrant you are in, all you really have to know at that point is the ICER. The problem arises because some points in the north-east quadrant will have the same ICER as points in the south-west quadrant, where in fact the points in the north-east quadrant will have positive incremental net health benefit and the south-west points will have negative INHB. With ICER you cannot boil everything down to one number.

How would one actually use this concept in cost-effectiveness analysis? Its advantages are that the units are those of effectiveness, or of currency if you prefer to use a monetary benefit, and these are readily understandable. Statistical inference is straightforward, as Andy Willan showed, because you are just taking linear combinations of things. Even the difficulties of censored data can be overcome with whatever estimation procedure suits your data. Then you can easily combine Andy Willan's 'five numbers' into the statistical inference for the INHB. This gives an unambiguous ranking of the points, by the INHB.

What is often put forward as a problem with this concept is that we do not know the correct λ, but I would suggest that the correct λ is the shadow price. An insurer who does not know his shadow price needs to find it out, because that is really where the competition is. For example, consider an older person whose children are grown up and who is approaching the stage where chronic disease is starting to loom. Maybe his health is good now but some of his friends and relatives may be developing cancer or diabetes or heart disease, and he is concerned that he might get sick before too long. Such a person might prefer to purchase insurance from a company that offers a plan that has a very high INHB. He wants to make sure that if he does get sick the doctors will be able to use all the latest technology in his treatment. Whereas somebody who is younger, healthier, maybe has children who are in good health, might prefer an insurance plan that has a lower INHB and hence a lower premium to be paid. He does not need to buy a more expensive insurance plan which guarantees to cover high-dose chemotherapy for breast cancer and all the expensive interventions that may be only slightly better than standard ones.

Let us say we have collected some data from a clinical trial and we are trying to present it in a way that accounts for the fact that different players may have different λ values. One insurance company may offer a de luxe package of insurance while another is offering a less expensive package that will substitute generics more freely, and so on. We want to analyse the data and present the analysis for both of those people. Fortunately it is not difficult. Stinnett and Mullahy (1998) originally proposed calculating intervals – be they confidence intervals or Bayesian intervals – for a range of values of λ, and then presenting those. Ben Van Hout and colleagues (1994) proposed several years ago plotting what we now recognise as the probability that the INHB is positive as a function of λ. He called it the acceptability curve. It had a slightly different interpretation when he first proposed it, but we have since recognised that this is just the Bayesian probability that the INHB is greater than zero, plotted as a function of λ. So a user of this information can look at these pictures and ask 'what is the interval estimate for INHB for the λ that I am aiming for?' If at that level of willingness to pay (λ) the interval indicates a positive INHB then, that treatment is something that the insurer would want to include in his plan. Conversely, if the interval lies entirely below zero at a particular λ value, then the insurer would not want to offer that treatment. It will depend on the λ value. The uncertainty will depend on the λ and also the interval will depend on λ, so insurers will have to decide on their own relevant shadow price, λ.

INHB from the perspective of an individual physician or a consumer is a totally different matter. But from the standpoint of an insurance company marketing its insurance plans as being optimal in some sense, it makes a lot of sense to think about it this way; not with kinked isoboles, as some have suggested, but with straight lines.

There is one more comment to make about the net benefit approach. Many people are unhappy with the south-west quadrant because in effect it represents selling health care, i.e. adopting an inferior but less costly treatment. But we presume that the insurer starts from the position that the object is to provide the greatest health benefit possible. So by saving money using a less expensive treatment without sacrificing too much health benefit, and applying that money somewhere else where it will do more good, presumably buying some other treatment that has a positive net health benefit, the total benefit can be increased. Of course an individual who has, say, cancer, would rather a more expensive treatment was adopted for his disease even if the money could be better spent elsewhere, say, in treating people who have diabetes. But for an insurer, either a public or private insurer, that in principle is what will govern rational behaviour in the long run.

So far this paper has been about what to estimate; let us now turn to how to estimate it, particularly about modes of inference. Reference has already been made to Bayesian inference, which has many different possible manifestations. The one espoused here is something one might call subjective inference. That seems a much better name for it, saying that each individual summarises the data, according to Bayes' theorem, given his own prior distribution over the unknowns. Probability distributions are used to summarise uncertainty about parameters in models or about future quantities that one is trying to predict; and hypotheses are evaluated by calculating posterior probabilities. In my view, that is what Bayesian inference means.

Compare that to frequentist inference, which says that we are going to fix the parameters – even though we do not know their values – and evaluate the properties of procedures in repeated samples. We will then use the procedures that have the best properties. There is a wide range of properties that one could look at, and of course one might be concerned about performance under a range of different assumptions about the process generating the data, and so on. It is not a trivial matter to decide what properties one should emphasise in a particular situation.

Now a major problem with frequentist inference is that it is really restrictive when it comes to interpreting data. You cannot make inferences without stating what your intentions were with respect to the design and analysis of the study. Compare this with Bayesian inference, which gives you more flexibility and freedom: you use the posterior distribution on the parameters to calculate the probabilities of the hypotheses are that you are interested in, however the study was designed. You cannot really do that in frequentist analysis, which I think gives a considerable edge to the Bayesian approach. This is important in cost-effectiveness studies, where costs are changing, new information is arising, you may want to synthesise data from different studies, and so on. There is just no provision for this in frequentist statistics.

Let me give a brief example of how one might implement a Bayesian analysis. This is not intended as an example of an ideal Bayesian analysis, in which one would have to carefully determine prior distributions, or perhaps assess the sensitivity of conclusions across a range of prior distributions. It is intended rather to give a sense of the quantities that can be computed in a Bayesian analysis, and how they would be interpreted.

Table 4.2 shows a summary of data from a trial comparing interleukin-1 receptor agonist (IL1ra) with placebo in the treatment of sepsis (Gordon et al. 1992, Fisher et al. 1994). These are not the original data but a summary I gleaned from other papers that discussed the data (Laska et al. 1997, Van Hout et al. 1994). The cost data are given in Dutch guilders (DFl).

Table 4.2 **Data from a clinical trial in sepsis**

	IL1ra	Placebo
Mean cost (DFl)	35,100	33,720
Var(mean cost)	4,000	4,000
Survival at one month	0.84	0.56
Var(survival rate)	0.09	0.09
Cov(survival, cost)	0.34	0.34

From straightforward calculations we get a z statistic for cost of 0.24 ($p = 0.81$), and a z statistic for survival of 2.20 ($p = 0.023$). Thus the IL1ra does not cost substantially more and seems to confer a considerable, and statistically significant, survival advantage. How then shall we evaluate cost-effectiveness?

Figure 4.2 **Joint posterior probability density of effectiveness and cost differences: comparing IL1ra to placebo**

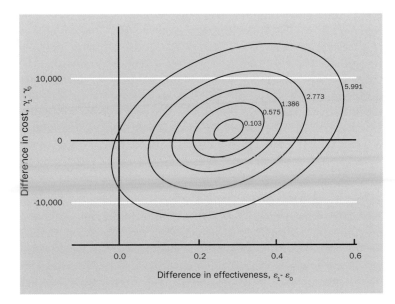

Figure 4.2 is a graph of an approximation to the joint posterior density of the effectiveness and cost differences, which is plotted on the same axes as the cost-effectiveness plane. The contours, from the centre outward, enclose 5%, 25%, 50%, 75% and 95% of the probability respectively. For this analysis we have assumed a flat, independent prior for cost and effectiveness differences, which is unlikely to agree with any actual prior but, given the moderate size of this dataset, should be a fair approximation to all but rather highly concentrated priors.

In a Bayesian analysis, we evaluate a hypothesis by its probability under the posterior distribution. Calculation using the prior in Figure 4.2 gives 59.4% probability to the north-east quadrant (cost-increasing trade-off), 0.3 % to the north-west quadrant (placebo dominates), 0.9% probability to the south west quadrant (cost-reducing trade-off) and 39.5% probability to the south-east quadrant (IL1ra dominates). Thus we can be quite certain that IL1ra increases survival, but it appears to have little effect on cost.

Van Hout et al. (1994) proposed to summarise uncertainty about cost-effectiveness with the cost-effectiveness-acceptability curve. Although they considered a different interpretation, one can think of the acceptability curve as a plot of the probability that the new treatment is cost-effective (has a positive INHB) as a function of the cost-effectiveness trade-off value λ. Figure 4.3 presents the curve for the sepsis data. The dotted line in this figure is at 95%, suggesting that the probability that IL1ra is cost-effective exceeds 95% for any insurer whose λ exceeds about DFl 40,000 per survivor. Thus insurers whose λ is low, say DFl 20,000 per survivor, would be less convinced of the value of IL1ra.

In an earlier paper (Heitjan et al. 1999b) we proposed to address the ambiguity in ICER interval estimates by computing 95% Bayesian probability intervals separately within the north-east and south-west quadrants. These intervals, together with more standard Fieller's method confidence intervals, are presented in Table 4.3. The Bayesian north-east interval has the interpretation that there is a 95% conditional posterior probability, given that IL1ra is more effective

Figure 4.3 **Cost-effectiveness acceptability curve, comparing IL1ra to placebo**

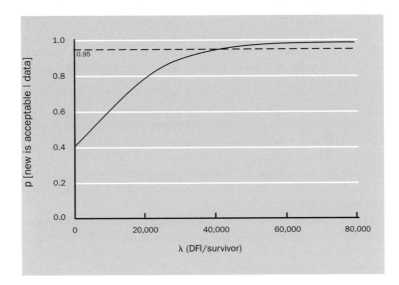

Table 4.3 **Interval estimates of ICER from the sepsis data**

Method	Confidence set (DFl/survivor)
Bayesian (NE quadrant)	(791, 63,400)
Bayesian (SW quadrant)	(8,400, 4,580,000)
Fieller (95%)	(-108,400, 55,900)
Fieller (98%)	(-∞, 135,200) ∪ (324,600, ∞)

and more costly than placebo, with the corresponding cost per survivor lying between DFl 791 and DFl 63,400. The SW interval has the interpretation that there is a 95% posterior conditional probability that the cost saving per life foregone is between DFl 8,400 and DFl 4,580,000. The Fieller 95% interval spans the range –DFl 108,400 to

+DFl 55,900. It is difficult to know how to interpret this because it contains both positive and negative numbers, and moreover the positive ratios have different interpretations in the north-east and south-west quadrants. Note that the Fieller 98% confidence set is actually the exterior of an interval. This occurs because the effectiveness difference is not significant at the 2% level. It is more difficult still to know how to interpret this.

To summarise the main points: first, I believe that the ICER has some role in cost-effectiveness analysis but that in most cases it is not an appropriate target for statistical estimation. The INHB resolves the ambiguities of the ICER approach and is straightforward to estimate. There is no single value of l that is relevant to all parties, but this is an essential element, not a disadvantage, of the INHB approach. Moreover, I believe that the Bayesian mode of inference has advantages over the frequentist mode of inference in estimating cost-effectiveness. Although in many situations the two modes give answers that are practically indistinguishable, one must always bear in mind the interpretation of the estimate and when one does so the difference is more than academic.

Finally, a little speculation about the future of research in this area: in their chapters, Andrew Willan and George Carides discuss modelling more complex data structures such as censored data. This is an important direction. Most of the methodological work published in this area so far has assumed that there is a simple, uncensored cost and effectiveness datum for each person in the study. But many clinical trials of chronic diseases have survival as the major endpoint, and in most studies the survival variable is potentially censored, in the sense that when the study ends some of the participants are still alive. For these subjects you do not know the survival time, just that it is greater than their survival so far. When survival is censored, then health care costs are censored too and one needs to account for this in the analysis to avoid bias. So the methods that Willan and Carides describe are important and are the logical next stage in this development.

Some examples of nonparametric modelling are presented in this book, in the sense that both Willan and Carides describe estimation of the survival curve or cumulative distribution of cost directly, without the aid of parametric statistical models. Often one can gain some efficiency of estimation, not to mention scientific insight, by using parametric models. This idea is somewhat out of vogue in biostatistics, but I believe that there continues to be value in parametric models, provided one subjects them to appropriate scrutiny in the model fitting process.

REFERENCES

Fisher C.J., Slotman G.J., Opal S.M. et al. 1994, 'Initial evaluation of human recombinant interleukin-1 receptor agonist in the treatment of sepsis syndrome: a randomized, open-label, placebo-controlled multicenter trial', *Critical Care Medicine*, 22, pp.12-21.

Gordon G.S., Fisher C.J., Slotman G.J. et al. 1992, 'Cost-effectiveness of treatment with interleukin-1 receptor agonist (IL-1ra) in patients with sepsis syndrome', *Clinical Research*, 40, 254A.

Heitjan D.F., Moskowitz A.J. and Whang W. 1999a, 'Problems with interval estimates of the incremental cost-effectiveness ratio', *Medical Decision Making*, 19, pp.9-15.

Heitjan D.F., Moskowitz A.J. and Whang W. 1999b, 'Bayesian estimation of cost-effectiveness ratios from clinical trials', *Health Economics*, 8, pp.191-201.

Karlsson G. and Johanneson M. 1996, 'The decision rules of cost-effectiveness analysis', *Pharmaco Economics*, 9, pp.113-120.

Laska E.M., Meisner M. and Siegel C. 1997 'Statistical inference for cost-effectiveness ratios', *Health Economics*, 6, pp.229-242.

Stinnett A.A. and Mullahy J. 1998 'Net health benefits: a new framework for the analysis of uncertainty in cost-effectiveness analysis', *Medical Decision Making*, 18, pp.S68-S80.

Van Hout B.A., Al M.J., Gordon G.S. and Rutten F.F.H. 1994, 'Costs, effects and C/E-ratios alongside a clinical trial', *Health Economics*, 3, pp.309-319.

Chapter 5
Bayesian sample size calculations

TONY O'HAGAN[1]

The subject of this paper is the problem of sample size estimation for cost-effectiveness analysis, and the Bayesian approach to this problem. The Bayesian approach is essentially as easy to implement as the standard frequentist calculations, while giving a little more insight and flexibility than the standard frequentist approach.

Consider this problem: a trial is to be designed to compare two treatments. Both efficacy and cost will be measured for each patient in the trial. How many patients should there be in each arm of the trial? Typically it is assumed that equal numbers of patients will be recruited to each arm, but this does not have to be the case. Nevertheless in this example we follow convention and present the same number of patients for each treatment; call this n.

We will judge cost effectiveness by the net monetary benefit, $\beta(K)$, of switching from treatment one to treatment two, defined as

$$\beta(K) = K \cdot \Delta_e - \Delta_c$$

where Δ_c is the true cost difference between the two treatments and Δ_e is the true effect difference. What we are basically interested in is whether $\beta(K)$ is positive, in which case treatment two (the new treatment) is more cost-effective than treatment one (the control).

The above formula emphasises that the net benefit is a function of K, which represents what the health care provider is prepared to pay for health gain. This can apply to the National Health Service provider or to insurers; we can refer to them in general as health care purchaser. K represents what the health care purchaser is prepared to pay in order to obtain an increase of one unit in efficacy. I use K rather than the commonly employed λ for this quantity since in statistics Greek letters tend to be reserved to represent unknown parameters, and the

---

[1] The author gratefully acknowledges the assistance of John Stevens of AstraZeneca Research and Development, Charnwood, England.

willingness to pay is not an unknown parameter in the sense of something to be estimated from the present analysis. Note that K must be specified, that is, you have to specify what the trade off, or exchange rate, is between the two value measures: money and health. Since the sample size will also depend on K, it has to be specified at the design stage of an evaluation – although varying K will show how the sample size varies as a function of the willingness to pay.

There are two stages to the study, the design stage and the analysis stage. Sample size calculations have to be at the design stage, before the data are collected. Statisticians should be involved at both the design stage and the subsequent analysis of the data stage, i.e. right at the beginning and right at the end of the trial. Note that if you are a frequentist statistician and you are worried about interim analysis, you must not let the statistician get involved in the middle – very strange!

When we get the data and do the analysis, we are seeking to prove in this case that the net benefit of the new treatment is positive. The desired outcome is to be able to report a probability of at least ω that treatment one is more cost-effective than treatment two. What this probability standard is will depend on whether you are a Bayesian or a frequentist, but in both cases you have a standard of proof that you are aiming for at the analysis stage. The design of the study will determine whether we have enough data to reach the standard we set for the analysis objective. We want to have a good chance, say δ, of being able to report the desired outcome. So there are two criteria: when we do the analysis, what sort of standard of proof do we want to set up; and when we design the study, how confident do we want to be that we are going to be able to reach this standard?

Hence there are two probabilities in this problem: ω, the standard of proof in terms of how confident we are in the differences between the treatments; and δ, the confidence with which we expect to achieve this standard of proof.

From a frequentist point of view the analysis objective will be formulated as follows. We wish to reject the null hypothesis of no net benefit at the $100(1 - \omega)\%$ level of significance. So a large ω will correspond to a good result since it will correspond to a small significance probability: for example $\omega = 0.95$ corresponds to the usual 5% significance test.

The Bayesian formulation is somewhat different. Bayesians will want to have at least a $100\omega\%$ posterior probability that $\beta(K)$ is positive. So the Bayesian has a much more direct statement at the end of their analysis. Instead of saying "I'm going to reject the null hypothesis at the 5% level of significance", the Bayesian says, "I am 95% sure that this treatment has a higher net benefit, or has a positive incremental net benefit". Put even more simply: "I am 95% sure that the treatment is better". For both Bayesian and frequentist, however, the analysis objective is to specify the value, 95% in this case, which serves as the standard of proof.

The design objective in the frequentist framework is the power calculation. The frequentist says: "I want a sample size large enough so that for some particular assumed true value of net benefit (the frequentist has to assume a value for the alternative hypothesis) I can be 80% sure of being able to get a significant result". This is the frequentist power calculation with $\delta = 0.8$.

The Bayesian statement is different in an important way. The Bayesian says "I want to have an 80% chance of being able to demonstrate that net benefit is positive". The crucial difference is that the Bayesian is not assuming any particular value for the 'true value' of $\beta(K)$. The Bayesian does not have to make an assumption about what the true value is because he averages over the prior distribution instead. This will be explained in more detail below.

At the analysis stage the frequentist and Bayesian objectives are rather similar, particularly if we use non-informative prior distributions. In general, in simple problems, a Bayesian analysis with a non-informative prior, a weak prior specification, will correspond pretty closely to a standard frequentist analysis. In that case the significance probability will probably be very similar to a Bayesian posterior probability. So at the analysis stage the alternative presentations are going to be pretty much the same.

In fact most people interpret the frequentist statement in a Bayesian way. They say "I've rejected this null hypothesis at the 5% level", meaning "it's 95% sure to be false". They always interpret things in the Bayesian way because that is what they want to be able to do: Bayesians always answer the question, while frequentists do not!

At the design stage, however, the frequentist and Bayesian objectives are quite different. The frequentist approach *fixes* the parameters at more or less arbitrary values. In fact the frequentist has to pretend that he actually knows what is going on exactly. By contrast, the Bayesian accepts that there is uncertainty about the true state of the world, and instead attempts to model this uncertainty through prior beliefs. So the Bayesian objective requires a probability δ of the desired analysis outcome *averaged* over the prior distribution of the parameters. When we put the two stages together, the frequentist makes a statement such as "we wish to have 70% power to reject the null hypothesis that $\beta(K) = 0$ at the 5% level, if the true value is say, $\beta(K) = £2,800$". The Bayesian statement is shorter "we wish to be 70% sure of obtaining a 95% posterior probability that $\beta(K) > 0$".

I firmly believe that everybody is naturally a Bayesian unless somebody has got at them and taught them something else. When advocating a Bayesian approach as I do, we have got to think about the prior distribution and for many people this is a stumbling block.

Various possibilities come to mind as to how you would formulate the prior distribution. A pharmaceutical company or a device manufacturer trying to set up a trial will naturally use the knowledge and beliefs they already have, perhaps from earlier trials. Alternatively, a trialist might want to take a broader view than that of the company that is trying to market the product, in which case they would seek out some more sceptical opinions from the wider community. There is also the possibility of using non-informative prior information; put simply: "I'm not going to use my prior because it gets me into trouble". Or, taking a totally sceptical view, one could start from the belief that the drug or device is actually harmful, and try to prove otherwise. For example, in the UK framework, if we are trying, say, to persuade the National Institute for Clinical Excellence (NICE) that a particular treatment is cost-effective, it would be interesting to use their prior information. After all, NICE should have some prior beliefs (otherwise why would the treatment be under consideration?) and these should be used when NICE is making its judgements. This prior information should somehow be representative of the community's views about treatment, or at least of informed people's views.

So while there is a whole range of things that we might do in relation to specifying prior information, these are not appropriate to the same degree at the two stages of the study. At the analysis stage, when I am trying to present a case to somebody else, to accept my drug or my new device or my new procedure, then I probably do not want to use my views about it, because they might be seen to be prejudiced. So there is a question mark about whether I want to use the company's opinion and there is also a question mark about whether I want to use the community's opinion. At the analysis stage we might even be persuaded that regulatory bodies should be using a non-informative or a sceptical prior.

However, at the design stage it is a totally different story. At this point I need to have my own beliefs about what is going to happen in this trial. It is impossible to design anything if you have no prior information. So a non-informative prior approach to the design stage is simply not an option. In fact, the frequentist approach to sample size calculation is based on exactly the opposite of what is known. The frequentist at the design stage is pretending to know the true parameters underlying the power calculation, and so assumes that the true value of $\beta(K)$ is known with certainty.

So in the Bayesian approach we are going to allow different prior distributions at the two stages: design and analysis. At the design stage the study will be set up based on my best knowledge about what is going to happen when I run this experiment. However, it is set up in such a way that at the analysis stage I am going to use a different prior distribution − the one that I am going to use to try and persuade people with. So the analysis prior will typically be non-informative, sceptical, perhaps some kind of consensus opinion of a community. Whereas the design prior should definitely be based on the best knowledge I can find − what it is that I actually believe.

To illustrate the Bayesian approach I will present a simple example, and then try to explain again why the Bayesian approach is different and gives you a rather more helpful answer than the frequentist approach. Briggs and Tambour (1998) presented a frequentist analysis based on the following hypothesised true values of cost and effect differences between the two treatments of $\Delta_c = 1,200$ and $\Delta_e = 0.8$ respectively. Setting K at 5,000 gives the hypothesised true net benefit as $\beta(K) = \beta(5,000) = 2,800$. They set a 5% two sided test, 70% power and they came up with equal sample sizes of 762 using a standard frequentist sample size calculation.

Now we employ a Bayesian formulation using a non-informative analysis prior. That is, at the analysis stage we are going to do essentially the same as a frequentist. Therefore we are designing with exactly the same objective at the analysis stage, but at the design stage we put a prior distribution on the expectation.

Typically when we go into these sorts of trials we may very well have a reasonable idea about what the effects or efficacy improvements will be from the results of other experiments. At this point, we probably know much less about how the costs are going to work out, so the costs start out being much more uncertain. People often talk about the problem of setting up these sorts of trials, and say that trying to prove cost-effectiveness is more difficult because costs are more variable. But the problem is not only that, it is that you start with so much less knowledge about what costs are going to be. That is what is really contributing to this large variance or standard deviation.

In this Bayesian example we set $\omega = 0.975$ because we are going to use a one sided test and $\omega = 0.975$ equates to a two-sided test with $\omega = 0.95$. We set δ to 0.70, but note that although this corresponds to the frequentist δ, this is a different 70% to the 70% power, because the design objective for the Bayesian framework is different. Working this Bayesian power calculation through generates equal sample sizes of 1,048 for the trial.

The reason why we end up with a larger sample size than with the frequentist approach is because of the different framework for the design stage. Figure 5.1 shows the design prior distribution for this problem with a mean net benefit at 6,800, but a large standard deviation, so in fact I only start with a probability of 0.774 that this will actually prove to be more cost effective (i.e. $p[\beta(K)>0] = 0.774$). This is important because this is what is used in the sample size calculation.

Figure 5.1 **Design prior for the cost-effective trial example**

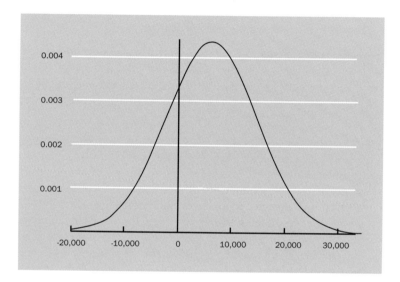

If we consider power for a moment, some power curves are shown in Figure 5.2. The lowest curve is a power curve for a small sample size, the middle one is for a moderate sample size and the top curve corresponds to a large sample size. What does the frequentist do? The frequentist fixes a particular value on the x-axis, say a net benefit of 2,800 from the above example, specifies a power level from the y-axis and finds where they cross in order to determine the sample size required. In terms of Figure 5.2 it is the sample size of 762 that is needed to get the power at 2,800 up to 0.7, which puts the frequentist somewhere between the top and middle curves.

Figure 5.2 **Power curves for three different sample sizes**

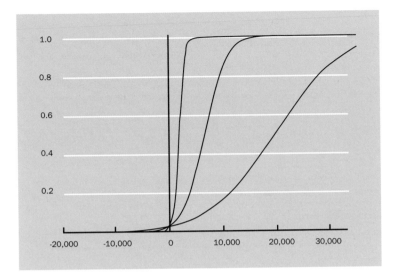

However, in the Bayesian framework we put these two things together, as shown in Figure 5.3. Instead of fixing a value on the x-axis and then trying to get the right power, we average the powers with respect to the prior distribution. That is, we calculate the average power for each of these curves with respect to the prior. You can see that the average power for the lowest power curve is going to be very low, because most of the time where we expect $\beta(K)$ to be, there is low power. The expected power averaged across the prior for each power curve gives the Bayesian analogue of the power calculation and can be termed the *assurance* of getting the desired outcome.

For the lowest power curve in Figures 5.2 and 5.3, the Bayesian expected power or assurance is just 0.15, for the middle curve this rises to 0.49 and for the top curve the assurance is 0.70. This is the prior probability for getting the desired result. We have had to go to a larger sample size in the Bayesian analysis in order to get the Bayesian assurance figure of 70%. However, the frequentist analysis is

Figure 5.3 **Integrating the design prior and power curves: Bayesian assurance**

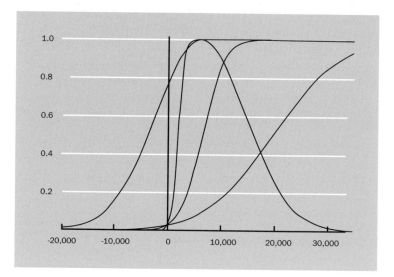

conditional – the frequentist only has their specified power level if the true state of the world is as they specified. The Bayesian on the other hand incorporates the overall uncertainty in the true state of the world and ends up with an unconditional probability, a 70% chance of showing the desired result.

In practical application of the frequentist sample size calculation, choices proceed with much ad hoc-ery and fiddling. Bayesians do not have to do this, they simply state what they believe and then design an analysis that gives a good chance of getting what they want. However, it is harder with this framework to get the same level of assurance. It is harder to get up to 70% because we cannot get past 77.4%, the original prior probability that the intervention is cost-effective. This original probability acts as a ceiling to the assurance level, which is why the Bayesian needs a greater sample size.

The Bayesian analysis has given a larger sample size, but it assures a 70% chance *overall* of demonstrating that treatment two will be more cost-effective than treatment one, partly because it recognises from the beginning that there is a good chance (100 - 77.4 = 22.6%) that treatment two is really *not* more cost-effective. The Bayesian approach allows considerable flexibility to represent the real problem because we do not then have to assume that we are going to analyse the data with a weak prior. After all, we may be designing this study for internal company purposes, maybe to persuade our boss, and therefore we might want to start with his prior. We can choose whatever we like for our prior beliefs at the analysis stage, and we can also choose our prior beliefs at the design stage, and fix the two criteria, ω and δ. The design objective is expressed as an overall assurance instead of requiring an assumed, more or less arbitrary, true effect. It says overall there is a 70% chance that the desired outcome will be proven, not that there is a 70% chance if the true state of the world coincides with your assumption, which we might think very unlikely. If we do not believe net benefit is exactly 2,800 what is the point of conditioning the sample size calculation on that?

In conclusion, I have tried to show that the Bayesian approach offers new insight into the problem of determining samples size for a cost-effectiveness trial, by clearly differentiating the analysis and design objectives. The method I have described then gives added flexibility by allowing different prior specifications at the design and analysis stage.

The two features together have allowed us to view the standard frequentist approach in Bayesian terms. The two approaches have similar analysis objectives and can be made to coincide at the analysis stage by setting a weak analysis prior. However, at the design stage the Bayesian design objective is in terms of assurance, which is quite different from the frequentist's power calculation. In essence assurance is expected power with respect to the prior distribution, but its value lies in the fact that we do not have to make an arbitrary assumption of a value for the true net benefit. The Bayesian and frequentist approaches can only be made to coincide at the design stage by adopting an unrealistically strong design prior.

Designing a trial with a given *assurance* of a positive outcome is more natural, and should be more useful to decision-makers, than the traditional power calculation.

REFERENCE

Briggs A. and Tambour M. 1998, 'The design and analysis of stochastic cost-effectiveness studies for the evaluation of health care interventions', *Swedish Working Papers in Economics*, No. 234. [Now published in: *Drug Information Journal* 2001, 35(4)]

Chapter 6
Methods for analysing censored cost data

GEORGE W. CARIDES[2]

The presence of censored observations in cost data collected alongside clinical trials poses a particular problem for economic analysis. In this paper, the problem of censoring is discussed together with some of the issues and challenges, both statistical and economic, of analysing censored cost data. A review of recently published methods for analysing censored cost data will be presented and a case study of a heart failure trial will be employed to illustrate and compare the methods. In addition to application of the methods in actual datasets, the results of a simulation study with respect to the performance of the estimators will be presented. The emphasis throughout is on the intuition behind the methods, keeping mathematical formulae to a minimum.

The general research question addressed here is: do patients who receive treatment A incur lower costs than those treated with B? Note, however, that it is very important to specify the time horizon over which costs are to be compared. Is it the entire lifetime of the patient, is it the follow-up period of the trial, or is it a fixed period within the trial? For example, are we interested in comparing the costs over five years of follow-up or over 10 years? In an ideal world, the clinical trial would be designed to address this economic research question with correspondingly large sample sizes, no missing data, and complete follow-up on all the patients (i.e. nobody would be censored).

In reality, this ideal case rarely exists. More commonly, a trial is designed to answer a clinical research question and the time horizon may be too short to answer the health economic question, whether that relates to cost or cost-effectiveness. The sample size may also be inadequate for precise estimation of the health economic endpoint(s)

[2] The author gratefully acknowledges the assistance of Joseph F. Heyse and John R. Cook, Merck Research Laboratories.

even though it might be adequate for the clinical endpoints. Typically, data are not normally distributed but highly skewed, include outliers, and exhibit a high degree of variability. There is also the potential for missing data and for incomplete follow-up or censored data.

Censored data usually occur when there is a staggered start date to a clinical trial. For example, a trial may last five years but not all patients enter the trial at the same time. For the patients who enter the trial early, complete five-year follow-up data may be available. But a patient who enters the trial six months prior to the trial's termination date and does not die before then only generates six months worth of cost data. This patient is censored with respect to the five-year cost of the treatment that is of interest.

It is worth distinguishing two situations that may arise in relation to the collection of the cost data. Sometimes we have the cost history available; i.e. we know when the costs occurred. For example, cost data may have been collected at monthly intervals. In other cases we may only know the total cost per patient; i.e. we may only know the cumulative cost at the time of death or censoring. The analytical methods that are appropriate will be dependent upon the type of data that are available. In many cases, it is not the cost data themselves that are captured but the level of resource utilisation, which requires an external price per unit of resource to be applied to generate a cost. So we may attach a price for a hospitalisation to each recorded inpatient episode or we may attach a per-diem cost to the recorded length of time that the patient was in hospital in order to generate a cost.

The clinical trial to be discussed as a case study is the 'Studies of Left Ventricular Dysfunction' (SOLVD). This was a randomised controlled clinical trial conducted with symptomatic heart failure patients who were randomised to either active treatment (enalapril) or placebo (SOLVD Investigators 1991). The clinical endpoints were mortality, hospitalisation and incidence of myocardial infarction. There were a total of 2,569 patients with a minimum of two years and a median of 2.9 years of follow-up. One goal of the health economic evaluation was to estimate and compare the three-year mean cumulative costs of the two treatments.

As is typically the case, the cost data were very right-skewed with variance increasing with greater survival time (heteroskedasticity). There was also evidence of a stratum dependent cost versus survival time relationship. Censoring was present with respect to both survival time and cost. A total of 22% of the patients, after three years, were censored in that they were followed for less than three years and had not died. If a patient had died and we observed the death, we would have the complete information on that person's cost. After death the cost would be zero.

It is very important when conducting an economic evaluation to conduct exploratory data analyses. Plotting the data in various ways can uncover features that may help to analyse and properly model the data. Figure 6.1 gives the simplest of plots: the frequency distribution or histogram of the total three-year cost for all the patients. This plot clearly shows the skewed nature of the cost data. Most cumulative

Figure 6.1 **SOLVD example – histogram of total 3-year cost ($US)**

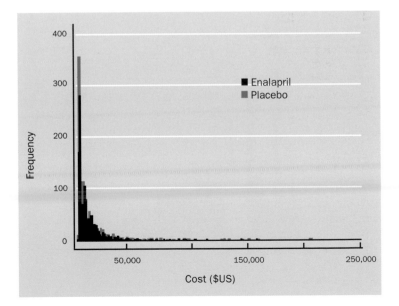

costs are concentrated below $25,000 but a few patients have much greater costs. The most expensive patient incurred over $200,000 after three years, while many other patients incurred only a few thousand dollars.

These kinds of data present problems in terms of usual normal theory assumptions, so it is useful to look at such data in a different way and perhaps uncover different features. Figure 6.2 presents a histogram of the same data after having taken the natural logarithm of the cost. We would not necessarily analyse the data on the transformed scale, but this plot does certainly point out some additional features. In particular, the figure reveals that the distributions are possibly bimodal, with patients separating into two main groups. In fact, an apparent bimodal distribution often indicates a mixture of two different distributions. For these data the difference is between those

Figure 6.2 **SOLVD example – histogram of log total 3-year cost ($US)**

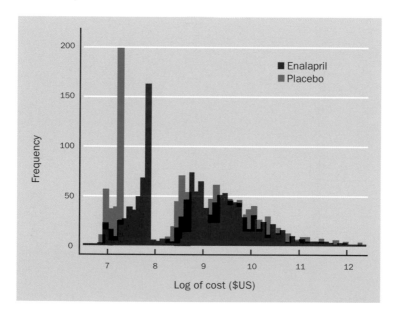

patients who were hospitalised prior to the end of three years and those who were not. The patients who were hospitalised incurred much greater costs than the patients who were not hospitalised. Among those not hospitalised, the Enalapril patients have higher cumulative costs because their cost includes the study drug cost.

Rather than simply looking at the univariate cost or transformations of it, it is also useful to look at plots of one variable versus another. In Figure 6.3, total cost after three years is plotted against follow-up time, with the plus symbol indicating censoring and a nought indicating death. The patients designated with a plus sign at three years were observed to be alive after three years of follow-up. Although in terms of survival they would be considered censored, in terms of cost they are complete because we are interested in the cost after three years of follow-up. A plus sign prior to year three indicates

Figure 6.3 **SOLVD example – total 3-year cost vs.**
survival time (years)

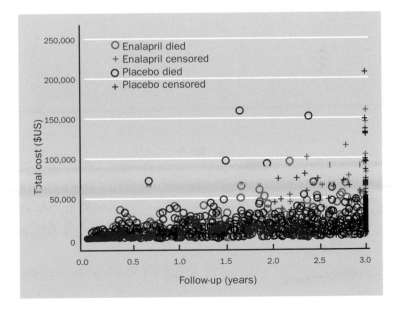

a patient for whom complete survival and cost were not available, i.e. who was censored for both survival time and cost.

If we can uncover some sort of relationship between the total cost and the time of death, we may be able to model that relationship in order to estimate the cost more efficiently. Thus we could obtain narrower confidence intervals and greater power for our task to detect differences between the treatment groups. However, it is not clear how we might use a regression model in this instance. A simple linear regression would be inappropriate given the degree of uncertainty as to the cost/survival time relationship and the dramatic increase in variability with greater follow-up time.

Consider Figure 6.4, which plots the log of the total cost versus follow-up time. Again the same split between patients who were hospitalised and those that were not is clearly in evidence. Here we

Figure 6.4 **SOLVD example – log total 3-year cost versus survival time (years)**

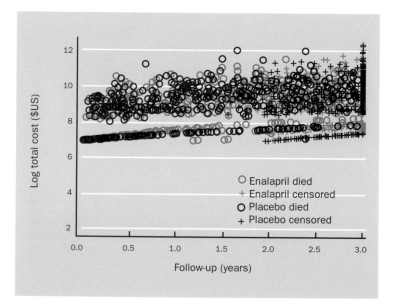

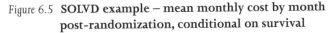

Figure 6.5 **SOLVD example – mean monthly cost by month post-randomization, conditional on survival**

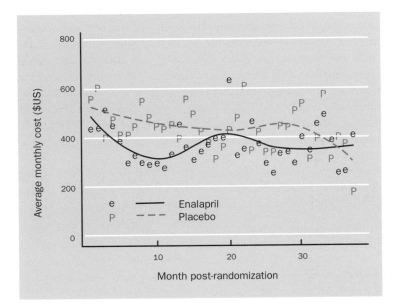

see much clearer relationships between cumulative cost and follow-up time for the patients who were hospitalised and those that were not hospitalised. This illustrates how sometimes we would want to make some sort of transformation, analyse the transformed data, and then back-transform.

Another way to look at the data is shown in Figure 6.5, which shows the mean monthly cost over time conditional on survival, together with a nonparametric regression or smoother fit to the data (Loader 1999). These nonparametric smoothers are very useful, not only to visualise data relationships but also to estimate the mean cumulative cost. Conditional on survival the enalapril group seems to have lower costs by month than the placebo group, even though the enalapril group includes cost of treatment while the placebo group does not. Again the explanation lies with hospitalisations: there were more hospitalisations in the placebo group than there were in the enalapril group; more than enough to offset the cost of the study medication in the enalapril group.

Our goal is to estimate and compare the mean costs per patient when information on cost for some patients is incomplete or censored due to follow-up times being less than the chosen time horizon of the clinical trial. So if the chosen time horizon is three years and a patient was followed for only six months, that patient is censored. A key question is whether patients' loss to follow up is covariate dependent. This is important because some of the methods are valid only if censoring is purely administrative, in which case hypothetical extension of the trial for enough time would result eventually in complete follow-up on all patients. However, if patients are dropping out of the study, say, because they are doing poorly, then the censoring mechanism is informative rather than administrative.

Several valid estimation methods exist for application to clinical trials where censoring is administrative (Lin et al. 1997; Bang and Tsiatis 2000; Carides et al. 2000; Strawderman 2000). For clinical trials where patients are dropping out due to some covariate-dependent reason, modification of these methods can be considered (Lin 2000). Further study is required, however, to assess the usefulness of such modifications in practice.

The focus of this chapter is on the case where administrative (i.e. uninformative) censoring exists. There are two general strategies for estimating the mean cost in this case. One class of methods is Inverse Probability Weighting (IPR), which is based on a strategy of weighting the costs more as more censoring occurs. The basic estimator, when cost histories are not available (i.e. we simply have a total cost per patient) is given by

(1) $\quad \dfrac{1}{N} \sum_i w_i C_i$

where N is the sample size, C is the total cost for the ith uncensored patient and w is a weight attached to the cost to reflect the proportion of censoring. In this estimate the total cost for each patient for whom there is complete follow-up is weighted proportionally to the amount of censoring at that time. Near the beginning of the study there will be very little censoring so the weight would be one or close to one. As time progresses and more censoring occurs, the costs of uncensored individuals are multiplied by a greater weight w_i. In effect, each uncensored patient has to represent others who were censored. So if the weight is three that means that a patient's cost has to represent himself plus two others.

The second version of the estimator can be used when cost histories are available. In this case, the data are partitioned into j time intervals and the estimator becomes

$$(2) \qquad \frac{1}{N} \sum_j \sum_i w_{ij} C_{ij}$$

where C_{ij} is the cost of the ith patient in the jth interval. In effect, the estimator (1) is computed for each interval and the sum is taken across the total number of intervals.

The other methods are conditional methods for censored data: conditioning cost either on survival or on death, multiplying by the probability of survival or death, and summing up. One published method to provide a way to estimate the mean cost under censoring (Lin et al. 1997) involves partitioning the full time period into intervals, perhaps years or months, depending on the nature of the cost data collected in the study. The average cost conditional on survival is calculated and then multiplied by the probability of survival. The method assumes that the censoring can only occur at interval cut points. So if the data on cost is available over years, and someone is lost to follow-up or censored in the middle of the year, then this method will contain some bias. We return to the Lin method later in the chapter.

A second method is one that I and colleagues have proposed and which we call the two-stage conditional method (Carides 1998; Carides et al. 2000). This method considers that total cost is comprised of survival time and error. Total cost is treated as the dependent variable and survival time as an independent variable, which has an impact on, or influences, the cost. This formulation acknowledges that simply knowing a person's survival time is not enough to determine the total cost precisely.

The mean cost is estimated in two stages. In the first stage, the average cost conditional on death is estimated – this is the regression component or the average cost given death. Here either a parametric regression model (such as ordinary least squares, possibly after some transformation) or a non-parametric smoother can be employed. The authors have found that in the biostatistics community, at least in the US, statisticians are reluctant to accept parametric regression models for estimation problems involving censored data. They have argued that the method may work well when the regression model is adequately identified, but that if the model were incorrectly identified the method would yield biased estimates. Therefore, we employed a non-parametric smoother, as can be seen in Figure 6.5, which shows the monthly costs over time together with a non-parametric fitted curve. The use of non-parametric regression allows us to utilise the information from the data without making strong parametric assumptions. Fundamentally, this is an issue for the analyst; if the analyst is confident that he has specified a parametric model that is reasonable then this can be used. Alternatively, the analyst may use a non-parametric smoother in situations where there is less confidence as to a reasonable model.

In the second stage, the probability of death at each one of those survival times is estimated. We employed the Kaplan-Meier estimator as a non-parametric estimator of survival, but the survival function could alternatively be estimated using a parametric model. The two-stage estimator may be expressed as

$$(3) \qquad \hat{\mu}_{TS} = \bar{I} + \sum_{j=1}^{k} \hat{g}_j(t_j) \{\hat{S}_j(t_{j-1}) - \hat{S}(t_j)\} + \bar{Y}_L \hat{S}(L)$$

where $\bar{I}$ is the sample average fixed initial, or start-up cost, $\hat{g}_j(t_j)$ is the estimate of mean total cost conditional on death at time t_j, $\hat{S}()$

is the Kaplan-Meier estimate of survival, and $\bar{Y}_L$ is the sample average cost of patients surviving to time L, the chosen time horizon for the study. The initial cost $\bar{I}$ does not depend on survival time and may include items such as diagnostic testing undergone just prior to entering the study.

In extensive simulation experiments, we have found efficiency gains from our method over the Lin method, which come about by exploiting the relationship between total cost and survival time. The Lin method essentially ignores that relationship. By exploiting the underlying relationship we can gain efficiency, i.e. reduce the variance. Other things being equal, we would like to have an estimator with lower variance over an estimator with larger variance. That gives us more precise estimates and greater power to detect possible differences between treatments.

Another advantage of our method is that it does not assume that censoring only occurs at interval cut points. Censoring can occur at any time. The method can also be extended to utilise the cost history where that is available, i.e. when we have information on the person's cost over time, not only at the time of death. Additional covariates other than survival time can be included into the model such as baseline patient characteristics. The form of the two-stage estimator which utilises the cost history is

$$(4) \qquad \hat{\mu}_{TSAS} = \bar{I} + \int_0^L \hat{f}(t)\hat{S}(t)dt$$

where $\hat{f}(t)$ is the estimated cost at follow-up time t conditional on survival to that time.

Table 6.1 shows a numerical example based on hypothetical data for 20 patients to illustrate how the simple weighted estimator (I) is calculated. Of the 20 patients, seven were censored prior to the time horizon of interest, L, which is 10 years. The goal is to estimate the 10-year mean cost. Seven of the patients are censored because they were followed for less than 10 years and they had not died. The remaining 13 are the patients whose costs we are going to utilise.

Table 6.1 **Estimation of 10-year mean cost – weighted estimator**

Patient number	Survival time	Censoring probability*	Weight (w)	Total cost (TC)	$w \cdot TC$
1	0.1	0	1	17,509	17,509
2	0.2	0	1	12,444	12,444
•	•	•	•	•	•
•	•	•	•	•	•
•	•	•	•	•	•
11	5.9	0.3	1.4	34,511	47,807
12	7.8	0.7	3.5	65,724	227,615
13	10.0	0.7	3.5	48,772	168,907

$$\hat{\mu}_W = (1/N)\sum w \cdot TC = 39{,}244$$

* Estimated by Kaplan-Meier, reversing the roles of censoring and death.

Patient number 1 was observed to have died at time 0.1 years. At that time the probability of having been censored was zero. The censoring probabilities are calculated using the Kaplan-Meier method, reversing the roles of censoring and death. That is, death is treated as a censoring event for time to censoring. At time 0.1 years the probability of censoring was zero, and so the weight we attach is 1. When we multiply the weight by the total cost of that patient we of course get back to the total cost of that patient, which means that patient number 1 is representing only his own total cost.

As we move towards increasing survival times the probability of patients being censored increases. For example, in Table 6.1 patient number 11 had a survival time of 5.9 years; the probability of being censored prior to that time was 0.3. So notice here that the weight has gone up, the weight is now 1.4 (the reciprocal of 1 - 0.3). See Bang and Tsiatis (2000) for the details of how to compute the weights. The point is to understand that as the amount of censoring increases the weight must go up so that the patients who were observed after that point can represent not only themselves but also some of the censored patients. In my example, for patient 11 we inflate their costs by 40%: they are representing themselves and 40% of somebody else. So it goes on: with increasing levels of censoring the weight increases.

When we sum up these weights times the total costs and divide by the number of patients we get our estimate of average 10-year costs using the weighted estimator of Bang and Tsiatis, namely $39,244.

Using the same data, we now apply the two-stage method. Figure 6.6 forms the basis of the first stage of the two-stage estimator. Plotted in the figure, for the 12 patients who were observed to have died prior to year 10, is the total variable cost: i.e. total cost less any initial or diagnostic cost that would be assumed to be fixed in that it would not depend on survival time. So variable cost in this context is related to survival time; there may be variation between patients in other costs, but if these are not related to survival time they are assumed fixed. The curve in Figure 6.6 is a non-parametric regression through these data. Non-parametric regression provides a method to estimate a relationship that is much more data dependent than an assumed parametric model.

Figure 6.6 **Total variable cost versus survival time with smooth fit (locfit*)**

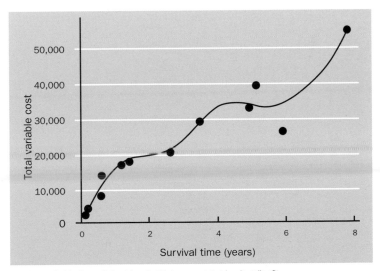

*locfit, available from: http://cm.bell-labs.com/stat/project/locfit

Based on this fit of the total variable cost, for each patient we can obtain the fitted variable cost and this is shown in Table 6.2. So for the patient with a survival time of 0.1 years, from the curve we have a fitted variable cost of $3,256. The second stage is to use the Kaplan-Meier estimate of the probability of death. The estimated probability of dying at time 0.1 years is 0.05. We then multiply the fitted variable cost by the probability of death, and do that for every patient, and then we sum up the resulting final column of figures. What we obtain is the average variable cost conditional upon death, conditional upon dying before 10 years, which in this illustrative example would be $23,144. If we now add to that the average fixed cost, i.e., in this example the average of the diagnostic costs, and also the average variable cost conditional upon survival to the end of the tenth year, we have obtained our estimator of the 10-year mean cost. We can see that although the methods look quite different, the resulting estimates are very similar; our two-stage estimate was $38,579 while the Bang-Tsiatis estimate was $39,244.

Table 6.2 **Estimation of 10-year mean cost – two-stage estimator**

Survival time	Fitted* variable cost (VC)	Prob. of death (p)**	VC·p
0.1	3,256	0.050	163
0.2	4,466	0.050	223
•	•	•	•
•	•	•	•
•	•	•	•
5.1	33,160	0.069	2,297
5.9	33,984	0.069	2,354
7.8	53,654	0.173	9,291
		$AVC|death = \sum VC \cdot p = 23,144$	

$$\hat{\mu}_{TS} = \sum AFC + AVC|death + AVC|survival$$
$$= 8,923 + 23,144 + 6,506$$
$$= 38,579$$

*locfit, available from: http://cm.bell-labs.com/stat/project/locfit
**Estimated by Kaplan-Meier.

The two estimators described above are the simple weighted estimator and the two-stage estimator. The weighted partitioned estimator is similar to the simple weighted estimator but we can utilise it when we have cost history information. Similarly, where we have information on cost over time for each individual patient we can utilise that information and partition our time period to get a partitioned two stage estimator that we refer to as two-stage AS, or average smooth, estimator. The two-stage method first averages the daily costs or monthly costs and then applies the parametric regression or smoother to these average costs. If we have information on cost over time, we can still apply the weighted and the two-stage estimators, but we can also apply the weighted partitioned estimator and the two-stage AS estimator. Table 6.3 shows these four methods applied to the SOLVD data example. The three-year mean costs are quite similar and all show a cost-saving for the enalapril arm of the trial compared to placebo. Note that the confidence intervals differ somewhat, reflecting differences in the variance properties of the estimators, which is discussed below.

With more than one method available for tackling a problem it is natural to want to see how well each method works in practice. It is not sufficient simply to apply each method to a single dataset since

Table 6.3 **Application of different estimation approaches to the SOLVD example – 3-year mean cost estimates ($)**

Method	Enalapril	Placebo	Δ	95% confidence interval
Weighted	11,324	12,898	-1,574	(-3,076, -263)
Weighted partitioned*	11,346	12,909	-1,563	(-3,242, 55)
Two-stage	11,201	12,931	-1,736	(-3,113, -317)
Two-stage – AS**	11,184	12,786	-1,602	(-2,920, -423)

*Based on yearly intervals.
**AS = 'average/smooth'.

there is no gold standard – the true mean cost is unknown. However, if we conduct a simulation study (sometimes called a numerical study, or a Monte Carlo simulation) we can specify the true mean that is to be estimated and then generate data which the different methods employ in order to estimate this mean. Repeating this process a large number of times lets us see how well the methods may do in practice.

In our simulation study, we set the task of estimating the 10-year mean cost where survival times are distributed according to the exponential distribution with an average survival time of six years. Censoring time is distributed uniformly from 0 to 12.5 years and as a result we have approximately 38% censoring prior to time 10 years. We have 100 patients and the total cost for each patient is made up of an initial diagnostic cost, annual variable costs and costs associated with death. We assumed that the costs would follow an autoregressive one (AR1) structure with year-to-year correlation varying from zero to one. The AR1 structure simply refers to how the costs vary from one year to the next. If the costs are positively correlated a patient with relatively high costs in the first year will tend to have relatively high costs in the second year, etc. If the patient had relatively low costs in the first year then they are likely to have relatively low costs in the second year and so on. Zero correlation would mean no correspondence at all between a patient's costs in successive years.

In order to compare the methods we ran 5,000 simulations, each time generating a data set of 100 patients, and estimated the mean 10-year cost using the four different methods. For each estimator we took the average across the 5,000 trials in order to provide an average figure for the accuracy of each estimator. The closer this average is to the assumed true mean, the more accurate the estimator. Zero would be perfect – i.e. there would be no bias in the estimator. As we diverge from zero, so we have bias. The farther away from zero we are the more bias we have. Other things being equal, we want an estimator with small bias. As can be seen from Figure 6.7, regardless of the correlation between costs over time from zero to one, the two-stage estimators seem to have lower bias than the weighted estimators. Although the bias is relatively small for all methods (less than 1% in

Figure 6.7 **Simulation study results: comparing the weighted and two-stage estimators**

Absolute value of percent relative bias

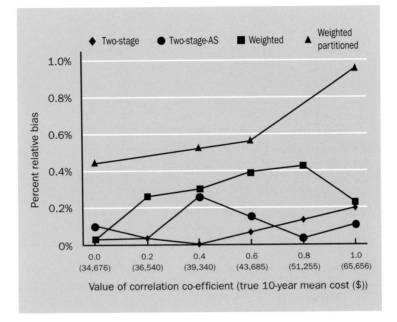

all cases), what is a little troubling is the apparent bias in the weighted partitioned estimator, especially as it seems to be higher for greater correlation.

As important as it is to have an estimator with low bias, it is also very important to have an estimator with low variance. Low variance is another criterion for judging the worth of an estimator. We desire an estimator that is not only very close to the true value of the parameter (in this case the mean) on average, but also has small variance or smaller variance than other possible estimators. An estimator that has relatively small variance is considered to be more efficient than other estimators and has greater power to detect differences in means.

Figure 6.8 **Simulation study results: comparing the weighted and two-stage estimators**
Percent relative efficiency (PRE) to weighted estimator

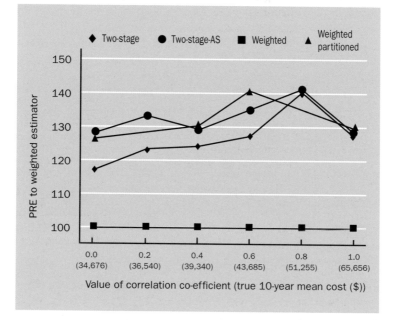

The simple weighted estimator was the least efficient of the four estimators: it had the greatest variance. Figure 6.8 shows the relative efficiency in percentage terms of the other estimators relative to the simple weighted estimator. In Figure 6.7, smaller values were better but in Figure 6.8 larger values are better. What we see is that the simple weighted estimator performs the worst, the two-stage estimator does much better, and the estimators which utilise the cost history – the weighted partitioned and the two-stage AS – perform better than the standard two-stage estimator.

Hence, where the cost history is not available, the simulation study suggests that the two-stage estimator performs better than the simple weighted estimator. Where information on cost is available over time it is preferable to employ either the weighted partitioned estimator or the two-stage AS estimator since these are more efficient. Although not shown in the figures, it is worth noting that the Lin estimator based on cost histories gives results comparable to those of the weighted partitioned estimator.

To summarise, the weighted and conditional methods are valid techniques for mean total cost estimation under administrative censoring. The simple weighted estimator and the two-stage estimator can be used when information is available only for total cost. Simulation results indicate that the two-stage estimator is more efficient that the simple weighted estimator, i.e. it has lower variance. If information is available on cost history, the forms of the estimators which utilise the cost histories generally perform better than those which do not. Intuitively this finding makes sense; because these methods utilise more useful information they should perform better. The simulation results suggest that the two-stage AS estimator is less biased than the partitioned weighted estimator especially when costs are highly correlated over time but more work is required to understand why this is the case.

Smoothing procedures such as local regression are very useful for visualisation and estimation when dealing with censored cost data problems. Smoothing procedures may be employed more often in this area since they provide us with an effective way to gain efficiency, and to estimate and visualise relationships without making strong parametric assumptions.

REFERENCES

Bang H. and Tsiatis A.A. 2000, 'Estimating medical costs with censored data', Biometrika, 87, 2, pp.329-343.

Carides G.W., Heyse J.F. and Iglewicz B. 2000, 'A regression-based method for estimating mean treatment cost in the presence of right-censoring', Biostatistics, 1, 3, pp.299-313.

Carides G.W. 1998, 'Estimation of mean treatment cost in the presence of right-censoring', unpublished PhD Dissertation, Temple University, Philadelphia.

Lin D.Y. 2000, 'Linear regression analysis of censored medical costs', *Biostatistics*, 1, 1, pp.35-47.

Lin D.Y., Feuer E.J., Etzioni R. and Wax Y. 1997, 'Estimating medical costs from incomplete follow-up data', *Biometrics*, 53, pp.419-434.

Loader C. 1999, *Local Regression and Likelihood*, New York: Springer-Verlag.

SOLVD Investigators 1991, 'Effect of enalapril on survival in patients with reduced left ventricular ejection fractions and congestive heart failure', *New England Journal of Medicine*, 325, pp.293-302.

Strawderman R.L. 2000, 'Estimating the mean of an increasing stochastic process at a censored stopping time', *Journal of the American Statistical Association*, Vol.95, No.452, pp.1192-1208.

Chapter 7
Estimating cost-effectiveness in multinational clinical trials

HENRY GLICK AND JOHN COOK[3]

When working with data from randomised trials and making policy decisions, there are many sources of uncertainty. Two of the most important sources of uncertainty surrounding the interpretation of the overall results of multinational or multi-centre trials are whether they apply to the countries and the centres that (i) participated in the trial; and (ii) did not participate in the trial. The focus of this paper is the first of these issues: whether the overall results of a multinational/centre study can be generalised to all the participating countries and centres in the study.

The generalisability issue addressed in this paper applies equally to generalisation from individual countries in multinational trials or from individual centres in multi-centre trials conducted in a single country, and to more complicated situations with centres embedded within countries. For example, in a multinational and multi-centred trial, a participating centre might be interested not only in whether the overall results apply in its particular country, but also whether they apply to itself. To simplify the explanation, this paper will discuss the applicability of multinational studies to participating countries, but in most if not all cases one could substitute the term centre for country and multi-centre for multinational.

There has been a growing concern that the pooled (or average) clinical and economic results for multinational trials may not be reflective of the results that would be observed in individual countries that participated in the trial. Some of the reasons why people are concerned about generalisability are that we might see differing morbidity and mortality patterns in different countries, different

[3] The authors gratefully acknowledges the assistance of Joe Heyse, Merck Research Laboratories, and Mike Drummond, University of York Centre for Health Economics.

practice patterns, different unit costs etc. In the face of all these types of variability that may affect the applicability of the pooled or average result to the participating countries, it may be difficult for decision makers in specific countries to draw conclusions about the value of the cost of the therapies that we are evaluating in the trials. This difficulty falls under the more general issue of generalisability, i.e. the applicability of the results of a given clinical trial to other populations or to sub-populations. In this paper, we propose statistical models to evaluate the homogeneity of the economic results among different countries (see Cook et.al., 2003).

Traditional approaches to generalising the economic results from multinational trials to individual countries include: (i) comparison of trial-wide clinical results with costs based on trial wide resource use together with unit costs from the country in question; and (ii) comparison of trial-wide clinical results with costs based just on the patients treated in that country. The problem with these approaches is that they ignore the fact that clinical outcomes and economic outcomes may influence one another. That is, differences in costs may affect practice patterns, which in turn may affect outcomes; and differences in practice patterns may affect outcomes, which in turn may affect costs. One of the alternatives to these two traditional approaches has been to use decision analytic models (see Drummond et al., 1992).

The impact of these different approaches can be seen in Table 7.1, taken from Willke et al. 1998, which shows data from a multinational study of tirilazad mesylate for subarachnoid haemorrhage in terms of cost per death averted. The results in the first column were obtained by multiplying each country's unit costs by the pooled resources use to estimate a cost-effectiveness ratio. Those in the second column were derived by use of the second approach outlined above. The treatment effect is taken from the trial as a whole but cost comes from the country-specific resource use and unit cost estimates. Some of the latter results differ substantially from those derived by use of country specific unit costs only. In country 5, we both save money and increase health giving a case of dominance; and in country 1 the cost

Table 7.1 **Impact of unit costs versus other variation**
Tirilazad Mesylate for subarachnoid haemorrhage, cost per
death averted (subanalysis using data from five countries)

Country	Trial- wide effects		Country-specific costs and effects
	Country-specific unit costs	Country-specific costs †	
1	46,818	5,921	11,450
2	57,636	91,906	60,358
3	53,891	90,487	244,133
4	69,145	93,326	181,259
5	65,800	**	**
Overall	45,892	45,892	45,892

Notes: † Country-specific resource use x Country-specific unit costs.
 ** New therapy dominates.
Source: Willke et al.1998

is very low leading to a low incremental cost-effectiveness ratio. In the
remaining three countries the ratio is substantially higher. So by using
both the countries' own costs and own resource use we have
effectively bifurcated the results into the two fairly good value
countries and the three countries where it may not be quite as
good value.

Notice what happens when we use country-specific effects as well as
country-specific costs, in the third column of Table 7.1. Now we
begin to see dramatic differences in the cost-effectiveness results
between countries. Of course, there are no indications of standard
errors in Table 7.1 and therefore it is not possible to judge whether
these observed differences are statistically significant. However, when
we recognise that countries can have different numerators and
different denominators, we have a more complete understanding of
the potential sources of heterogeneity or difference in the economic
outcomes associated with a new therapy.

More recently, another approach that some people have thought
might be appropriate for generalizing economic results is to test the

homogeneity of the cost and effect components of the cost-effectiveness ratio. That is, to test whether the treatment effect is the same across all the countries in the trial and test whether the cost difference is the same across all the countries. If we can convince ourselves that both the clinical effect and cost difference are homogeneous, then we might be tempted to assume that the cost effectiveness ratio is homogeneous.

The problem with the latter assumption is that a finding of homogeneity of a therapy's independent impacts on costs and outcomes need not guarantee the homogeneity of the resulting cost-effectiveness ratio. Statistical tests of clinical endpoints of trials are often based on relative measures such as odds ratios, hazards ratios or relative risks and most of our homogeneity tests for clinical endpoints are based on these relative measures. Economic outcomes, on the other hand, are a result of absolute differences, and cost-effectiveness ratios are computed as the ratio of absolute differences in cost and outcomes. Heterogeneity in absolute treatment effects measured as a difference can occur when there are large country-to-country differences in the underlying rate of events, coupled with homogeneity in the relevant treatment effects (i.e., a constant multiplicative treatment effect).

Table 7.2 **Illustrative example**

Country	$P_{control}$	Odds ratio	P_{active}†	Difference
Homogeneous odds ratios				
1	0.2	0.5	0.111	0.099
2	0.1	0.5	0.053	0.047
Heterogeneous odds ratios				
1	0.2	0.72	0.153	0.047
2	0.1	0.5	0.053	0.047

P_{active} = probability of death among those receiving active intervention.

$P_{control}$ = probability of death among those not receiving active intervention.

Difference = $P_{control} - P_{active}$

† $P_{active} = (P_{control} \times OR) / \{(P_{control} \times OR) + (1 - P_{control})\}$

where OR = odds ratio

A very simple, illustrative example is presented in Table 7.2. Suppose that the probability of death in the placebo group is 20% in country 1 and 10% in country 2, that is the health system in the first country does not do a very good job of treating the illness, while the health system in the second country does a much better job. In one case we assume that the odds ratio for death associated with active intervention is 0.5 and has been found to be homogeneous between the two countries. In an alternative case we assume that the odds ratios differ – in country 1 it is 0.72 and in country 2 it is 0.5 – and that this evidence of heterogeneity is statistically significant. The question is: in which case will the absolute difference in country-specific outcome be similar?

In the first case of homogenous odds ratios:

- in country 1 the control group had a 20% mortality and combined with an odds ratio for treatment of 0.5 gives a probability of death of 0.11 for the active treatment group;

- in country 2 with the baseline mortality of 10% the same odds ratios gives a probability of death of 0.047.

Despite homogeneity in the odds ratios between countries, many more deaths are averted in country one than in country two. This could clearly generate heterogeneity in the cost-effectiveness analysis by country.

In the second case, despite heterogeneous odds ratios the deaths averted are the same at 0.047 in both countries. In other words, the denominator of the cost-effectiveness ratios is going to be the same in both countries, yet statistically we had concluded that the treatment effect was heterogeneous. The main point of this example is that it is not clear that it would be a good strategy to test separately the homogeneity of the clinical effect and the cost difference in order to make judgments about the likely homogeneity of the cost-effectiveness ratio itself.

The complexities related to assessing the homogeneity of country-specific cost-effectiveness via independent assessment of the homogeneity of the clinical effect and cost differences suggests an alternative approach. Estimate country-specific cost-effectiveness ratios or net health benefits and evaluate their homogeneity directly. The more precise pooled estimate of cost-effectiveness (the ratio or net benefit) for the overall study would be used to represent the participating countries' results if: (i) it appears that there is no country by ratio (country by net benefits) interaction; and (ii) the minimum detectable difference was small enough to be economically important. In the example below, the focus of the analysis is on the homogeneity of net monetary benefits, since these have more desirable statistical properties than cost-effectiveness ratios. However, there are similar statistical techniques for ratios as well, so it is possible to do an equivalent analysis based just on the cost-effectiveness ratios

Gail and Simon (1985) have proposed two tests of homogeneity to determine whether the results of a study are inconsistent in both direction and magnitude or whether they are consistent in direction but not in magnitude. They defined a qualitative or cross-over interaction as one where the treatment effect is positive (i.e. cost-effective) in some countries and negative (i.e. not cost-effective) in others. That is, the cost-effectiveness between countries is inconsistent in both direction and magnitude. They defined a non-cross-over interaction as one where there is variation in the magnitude of the effect (i.e. cost-effectiveness) but not in its direction (e.g. when the treatment effect suggests an acceptable cost-effectiveness ratio in all countries). Peto (1982) has termed the latter a quantitative interaction.

A finding of qualitative interaction suggests the following relationships for the clinical outcome, for the costs and for the economic outcome:

- for the clinical outcome, the treatment is effective in some countries and ineffective in others;

- for the cost outcome, the treatment saves money in some countries and adds costs in others;

- for the cost-effectiveness results, the treatment has acceptable ratios in some countries and unacceptably high ratios in others; or in net benefit terms, positive net benefits in some countries and negative in others.

A finding of a quantitative interaction suggests:

- for the clinical outcome, the treatment is shown to be effective/ineffective in all countries, but differs in its degree of effectiveness/ineffectiveness;

- for costs, the treatment saves/costs money in all countries but differs in the degree of savings/costs;

- for cost-effectiveness, the ratio is acceptable/unacceptable (or the net health benefits are greater/less than zero) in all countries, but differs in its degree of acceptability.

In terms of estimation, the formal test for a qualitative treatment by country interaction of effects uses estimates of the treatment effect (net monetary benefit) and its variance for each of the countries being evaluated. The statistical test is based on a likelihood ratio, with critical values given in Gail and Simon (1985), and there is also a power test that has been described for qualitative interaction (Pan and Wolfe, 1997).

The test for quantitative interaction is based on the sum of squared errors on the country-specific treatment effects and the variance of those effects. For cost-effectiveness analysis, country-specific net monetary benefits and variance estimates are used to compute the test statistic. We use a weighted mean in estimating the errors rather than the arithmetic mean and the test statistic is compared to critical values of the Chi-squared distribution with one less degree for freedom than there are countries being evaluated.

An Example: The Scandinavian Simvastatin Survival Study ('4S') was a randomised double blind placebo controlled study of 4,444 patients that was conducted in five Scandinavian countries (see Scandinavian Simvastatin Survival Study Group, 1994). There was a wide range in terms of the sample sizes that were recruited to the study across these countries: in Iceland there were just 150 individuals, Denmark had 713, Finland 868, Norway had 1,025, and Sweden had 1,681. So there was quite a disparity in terms of the amount of information available in one country versus another. In this study patients were followed for a median of 5.4 years, but all patients were followed for five years, unless they had died. Hence the cost-effectiveness results in this example are based on five-year costs and five-year survival probabilities.

Figure 7.1, taken from Cook et.al.,2003, gives a sense of the basic results within each country. The y-axis shows the incremental cost for simvastatin relative to placebo ranging from zero up to $2,500 per patient. The x-axis shows the incremental survival probability ranging from zero up to 5%. The overall effect is marked with an asterisk and shows a gain in survival probability of 3.3% at an additional cost of just over $2,000 per individual. There is variation around these estimates as you look across the countries. Incremental survival is lowest in Iceland and highest in Denmark and Norway. Incremental cost is also lowest in Iceland and is greatest in Finland.

Figure 7.1 **4S: incremental costs and effectiveness (simvastatin – placebo)**

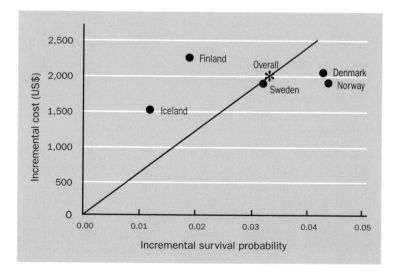

What we want to determine is whether or not there is qualitative or quantitative interaction here with respect to the cost-effectiveness of simvastatin in the individual countries. We could consider this question either in terms of cost-effectiveness ratios (represented by the slopes of the lines joining each point to the origin in Figure 7.1) or in terms of net benefits (essentially the minimum distances between the data points and a reference line representing the ceiling ratio that decision makers are willing to pay). Note that one needs to identify a threshold or ceiling ratio to judge whether an intervention is cost-effective or not cost-effective, whether cost-effectiveness ratios or net benefits are used.

If, for example, one compared the point estimates for the five countries to a ceiling ratio of $75,000 per additional survivor, one might conclude that in Iceland and Finland the product is not cost-effective, whereas in Sweden, Norway and Denmark, it is.[4] Such a comparison is problematic because it does not take into account the variability that exists within the estimates. If we use that ceiling threshold of $75,000 per additional survivor, we can estimate the net monetary benefit for each patient within this study by taking the $75,000 and multiplying it by one if they survived and zero if they did not and then subtracting out the cost of treating the individual. We can then take the average net benefit across individuals within a country for the two treatments, simvastatin and placebo, and see the difference between countries. Results of this calculation are presented in Table 7.3.

The results show that in Finland and Iceland we have negative estimates for the incremental net monetary benefit of treatment, whereas it is positive in Norway, Denmark and Sweden. The variability

---

[4] Given that the ceiling ratio is not well known in any country and is likely to differ between countries, then in practice it is desirable to test whether the results were homogeneous across a range of different ceiling ratio values. For example, in addition to testing with a value of $75,000 per survivor, the test could be repeated for a ceiling ratio of $50,000 per survivor, and for other values. However, do not use separate ceiling ratios in different countries in the calculation of a pooled result; use a common ceiling ratios across countries, but test at different levels of that ratio.

Table 7.3 **4S: net benefits ($): assessment of interaction**

Country	Net benefit Mean	S.E.
Denmark	1,208.8	1,964.7
Finland	-850.2	1,306.2
Iceland	-636.5	3,404.0
Norway	1,370.9	1,486.8
Sweden	542.3	1,105.7

Assuming $\lambda = \$75,000$ per survivor.

in Iceland is much larger than in the other countries, which reflects the small sample size. So the question is whether or not these apparent differences between countries are meaningful once the reduced sample size (and therefore increased variance) is taken into account. Applying the Gail and Simon test for quantitative interaction would suggest that the differences are not significant; in other words it is unlikely that the variability in the results of Table 7.3 reflects real differences among the different countries. Typically in these types of tests, because of the low power, we do not use a stringent test such as an alpha of 0.05 to judge whether or not interaction exists, rather we relax the test to an alpha of 0.2. Alternatively, Piantadosi and Gail (1993) have proposed another method for testing for homogeneity, based upon using confidence intervals, and this is the method that Pan and Wolfe (1997) used in order to assess the issues of power that are addressed below. So there is not one single way of going about assessing qualitative or quantitative interaction – the Gail and Simon test is just one approach that can be used.

Although the Gail and Simon method suggested that there was no interaction in our 4S example, the question is whether or not we are confident in those results in the light of the low power of the test. Another question has to do with the source of the lack of power: is it because there is so much variation in the cost from one country to the next, that we would have needed very large sample sizes in order to pick up differences between countries? In order to address these issues an ex-post power calculation was undertaken. It provides a sense of whether there was a chance of seeing any differences among the countries given the sample sizes that were available and given the amount of variation that was seen. Of course, the power also depends on the magnitude of differences to be detected – in a prospective assessment of power one would need to be able to quantify what is really an important difference in order to see whether or not you had enough power to pick up that difference.

Recall the pattern of the 4S results was that two countries, Iceland and Finland, had negative net benefits and that the other three countries had positive net benefits. Had we used these observed results as if they represented the true net benefit differences among the countries that we were trying to detect, then with an alpha of 0.05, we would have had no chance of identifying these differences as significant or concluding that there was qualitative interaction among those countries. But if we relax the alpha value to 0.2, indicating that we are more willing to come up with a wrong conclusion, then our power would increase to 12%.

Why is the power in this particular study so low? It could be due to sample size or to variability. With a sample of 4,444 individuals from five countries, the sample size does not seem particularly low, apart from in Iceland which clearly did have fewer patients (150) recruited. However, even if we exclude Iceland there is little increase in power. In fact it is in the variability of net benefits where it is most likely that the loss in power is occurring in this particular case.

The variability of net benefits comes from two components: the cost and the effect. Typically we might consider the cost component to be more variable, however in this case it is the differences in effects that contributes most to the variability in net benefit. Recall that the change in survival probabilities is multiplied by $75,000, so that survival probability is going to be very influential in terms of the variability of net heath benefits. If you evaluate the ratio of the standard errors of the health outcome effect side and costs in the five countries, it turns out that it is imprecision in terms of the estimate of survival probability that is leading to the large variability in the net health benefits. If the amount of variability in survival was equivalent to that of cost then the power of the test would be around 70%, and most people would be quite happy with power of that size. So here is an example where one needs a larger sample size, not to estimate cost, but because the variability on the clinical outcome is contributing most to the variability of the cost-effectiveness statistic of interest.

In this chapter we have outlined a method for evaluating the homogeneity of country-specific cost-effectiveness ratios or net monetary benefits calculated in multinational trials, to determine whether the pooled result is representative for all countries or whether it is more appropriate to report separate ratios for each country. In addition to a general test of interaction, we have proposed determining if the treatment effects are inconsistent in both direction and magnitude or if they are consistent in direction but not in magnitude. This set of tests is a reformulation of the Gail and Simons test for the evaluation of homogeneity of clinical outcomes to make it applicable to the homogeneity of economic results.

A finding of homogeneity is a necessary but not a sufficient condition for attributing the pooled results of the trial to all of the countries that participated in the trial. Given potential limitations in the power of a test of homogeneity, failure to detect heterogeneity does not mean the results are homogenous. Ex post power calculations provide additional information about the degree of homogeneity that may exist when heterogeneity is not detected. For example, if it turns out that there could have been $10,000 difference in net health benefits between the countries and we would still have concluded that they were homogenous, then the decision maker will not have learned much from our evaluation of homogeneity.

When there is evidence of heterogeneity, one should explore the possible reasons for it and determine whether it is qualitative or quantitative in nature. Use of pooled estimates to represent the cost-effectiveness ratio for all countries is less problematic in the presence of quantitative interaction, where all results are acceptable but of different magnitudes or they are all unacceptable but of different magnitudes, since the direction of the effect (cost-effectiveness acceptability) is the same in all countries. Thus if all decision makers use the same ceiling ratio, conclusions would not change for individual countries between using country-specific or pooled results.

In the face of qualitative interaction, pooled estimates should not be used. If you were to find qualitative interactions you need instead to investigate why the therapy is cost-effective in some countries and not in others.

Although the focus of this paper has been on generalisability across countries in multinational studies, the same techniques can be employed to assess homogeneity across practice patterns or across levels of illness or other sub-groups such as men and women. So we can use the evidence of heterogeneity to determine whether the pooled results of cost-effectiveness studies are applicable across countries, practice patterns, levels of illness severity etc.. We also may desire to know about cost-effectiveness in settings or populations that are unlike anything that is observed in the trial. But unless the trial has observed at least something like these settings it will not provide us with information to do that.

One common reaction to this problem is to say "the trial is not really representative so we should use a decision analysis approach". The problem with this approach, however, is that if we do not have any evidence of whether what was observed in the trial applies to one country versus another, where does the evidence for use in a decision model come from? If we did not have enough evidence in these trials to distinguish between the costs in different countries and effects in different countries, where is the modeller going to come up with the data to support the decision analytic model of whether the costs and effects are different between countries? So if it turns out, as is particularly likely with new medicines or other treatments that have not been used before, that the trial evidence is all the evidence we have, it is not clear that a decision analytic model provides us with a solution.

In conclusion, the growing policy demand for health technology assessment often requires that limited clinical and economic data be applied to a variety of different populations. Tests used to assess country by treatment interactions for clinical endpoints can be adapted to assess the presence of an interaction in economic outcomes including net health benefits and the cost-effectiveness ratio. The use of the Gail and Simon test for qualitative and quantitative interaction can be useful in determining if and how country-specific results can be pooled to obtain trial-wide estimates of economic impact. Tests of homogeneity should partially offset difficulties decision makers in specific countries have in drawing useful conclusions from multinational trials about the value of a therapy in their own specific country.

In future it will be important to consider design issues such as sample size per country when economic assessments are planned in multinational clinical trials. In our 4S example there were five countries and some of those countries had more than 1,000 patients entered in the trial. However, it is common for multinational studies to be conducted in 50 countries and maybe some of those countries contribute only 20 patients. You are not going to be able to use the estimates by country in those trials to assess generalisability. It may make sense in such situations to group particular countries − say Western European countries, developing countries, North America − and test the homogeneity across those categories to see if the trial-wide result appears homogeneous. But if we want to test it by country we are going to have to change the way we design some multinational clinical trials and pay more attention to the number of patients recruited in each country.

REFERENCES

Cook JR, Drummond M, Glick H, Heyse JF. Assessing the appropriateness of combining economic data from multinational clinical trials. Statistics in Medicine. 2003; 22:1955-76

Drummond M.F., Bloom B.S., Carrin G., Hillman A.L., Hutchings H.C., Knill-Jones R.P., de Pouvourville G. and Torfs K. 1992, 'Issues in the cross-national assessment of health technology', *International Journal of Technology Assessment in Health Care*, 8, pp.671-682.